D0669151

WHAT YOU NEED TO KNOW IF
EPILEPSY
HAS TOUCHED YOUR LIFE

A GUIDE IN PLAIN ENGLISH

AUTHOR
MARCELO LANCMAN M.D.

CONTRIBUTING AUTHORS
OLGICA LABAN-GRANT, M.D.
EVAN FERTIG, M.D.
LORNA MYERS, Ph.D.
DANA CASENDINO, R.D., C.N.S.C.

What You Need to Know if Epilepsy has Touched your Life
Copyright © Epilepsy Life Links Series
All rights reserved.
ISBN-10: 1475105312
EAN-13: 9781475105315
Library of Congress Control Number: 2012905652
Createspace, North Charleston, SC

TABLE OF CONTENTS

DEDICATION

THIS BOOK IS DEDICATED TO OUR PATIENTS AND ALL OTHERS WHO HAVE EPILEPSY. YOU ARE A DAILY INSPIRATION TO US.

INTRODUCTION

Epilepsy.

It's a unique disorder, characterized by seizures, uncontrolled waves of electrical activity racing through the brain – an "electrical tsunami" swamping the delicate tissue that controls every aspect of the body and mind, houses our memory and makes us one-of-a-kind.

It can be frightening because, like a tsunami, it can strike suddenly and powerfully, without warning.

And it's surprisingly common, afflicting some 2.5 million Americans.

But it's also manageable. In some cases, we can remove the source of epilepsy from the brain and banish it forever. And in other cases, we can do a great deal to keep it under control, prevent future seizures, reduce the severity of those that do occur, and ameliorate much of the physical and psychological impairment they cause.

We have made great strides in controlling epileptic seizures and improving the lives of those suffering from the disorder. I know this is true because I'm an epileptologist, a medical doctor who specializes in the treatment of epilepsy. In the 28 years that I've been in practice, I've worked with thousands of people, helping them learn to control the condition and reclaim their lives.

I've written this book so that you, like so many of my patients, can turn distress into success. Using the comprehensive treatment team approach we've developed at the Northeast Regional Epilepsy Group, there is a very good chance you can:

- Reduce the frequency and severity of your seizures, or even eliminate them entirely

- Overcome obstacles to daily living, and go from being afraid to leave your house to eagerly participating in life

- Combat psychological distress, turning depression and anxiety into optimism and hope for the future

- Break through the discrimination that may be holding you back

THE KEY BREAKTHROUGH

Over the past several decades, medical researchers have been developing newer and better medicines for epilepsy, giving doctors and patients stronger and more targeted tools for combating seizures. But the simple truth is that *medicines alone are often insufficient*. For approximately a third of patients, even the "right" medication can't control seizures. Of those who do gain control of their seizures through medication, there may be other problems like side effects, memory impairments, social difficulties and so on.

Epilepsy is a multi-faceted disorder that strikes both mind and body, potentially impairing physical function, memory, daily living and much more. There's no medicine that can "cure" all of these problems, even if it does keep the seizures under control. Still, most people with epilepsy are given medication alone, for many treating doctors are under the mistaken impression that this is enough.

Far from being *cured* with medication, epilepsy can be managed, but only if *all* of its causes, symptoms and associated problems are tackled as part of a broadly-based treatment and support program. Then and only then can a person with epilepsy reach her/his life fullest physical, psychological and emotional potential.

Obviously, it's very important to select the proper anti-seizure medication, one that can keep the "electrical tsunami" at bay or reduce the frequency and severity of attacks. But if you've ever seen pictures of the aftermath of a tsunami, you know that simply warding off the next one is only part of the job. There's still plenty of clean up and re-building of the infrastructure left to do. Unfortunately, the majority of patients are not given anything more than a prescription for anti-epileptic medication and some general advice. Frequently, they are not told that there's much more they can do to improve their lives.

WHAT YOU'LL LEARN...

In this book, you'll learn all about anti-seizure medications, then go beyond to learn how to raise your seizure threshold to make it even harder for a seizure to strike. That's like building a higher and stronger dam to make it harder for any new waves to splash over.

You'll learn about surgeries for epilepsy, experimental treatments, diet, alternative and complementary treatments. You'll find out about supportive treatments such as psychotherapy, memory treatment and support groups. And you'll learn how to live well with epilepsy, whether at work, during pregnancy, when you have a child with epilepsy, when playing sports or exercising and when handling epilepsy-related legal issues. There is also a chapter on coping strategies for family and friends of a person with epilepsy. In short, you'll learn how to manage every aspect of your epilepsy, from the physical to the psychological. And you'll be on the road to living a fuller and happier life.

As you'll see, epilepsy doesn't have to control your life. *You* can take charge of your epilepsy, and find ways to live a healthy, productive and fulfilling life.

CHAPTER ONE
EPILEPSY: A SURGE OF ELECTRICITY
TO THE BRAIN

It starts with some funny zigzagging lines that cut across your field of vision. "Uh oh," you say to yourself. "Here we go again." Then suddenly your left leg begins to jerk violently. You know what's happening: it's another seizure. A wave of panic hits you as you sink into the nearest chair and wait for the jerking to recede and finally fade away. A few minutes later (although it seems like hours), the seizure is over, leaving you exhausted and shaken.

If you were to look at a live human brain – touch it, poke it, examine bits of it under a microscope, even smell it – you would probably report that it's "squishy," it has areas with different textures and so on. The one thing you would probably *not* say is that it's electrically-charged, with currents constantly zipping from here to there in myriad patterns. Those electrical currents are key parts of the brain's communications system, making it possible for billions of cells to talk to each other, deliver status reports, and give and receive orders.

This electricity helps you move your left arm in a certain way at a particular time because a finely-focused electrical current carries the "move left arm" message from a very specific part of your brain at just the right moment. You're able to sit up in a chair as you read this, without even thinking about it, because numerous electrical currents deliver the proper messages to the parts of your brain involved in sitting.

Your brain is constantly "plugged in," which means that the electrical flow never stops and must be carefully controlled. If, for example, the "move left arm" electrical current becomes too strong, your arm will start flapping. And if an excessive amount of electrical current floods the areas of your brain dealing with awareness, you might "blow a fuse" and go blank for a few moments, or even longer.

Just as your house uses wires, switches, fuses, outlets and other devices to manage the flow of electricity through its walls, appliances, heaters and computers, the human brain has special structures and chemicals that control its electrical flow. As long as these are working well, the electricity will be sent to the right places at the right times, in just the right amounts. But should something go wrong ...

What if the electrical circuits in your car suddenly went wild and your horn started honking, your windows flying up and down and your sparkplugs firing at the wrong time? Or so much electricity raced through the wires in your house that your computer and TV were blown out, your blender went into high gear, and your AC kicked into overdrive and refused to stop?

Something similar happens inside a brain affected by epilepsy. If the areas of the brain governing sensations are zapped, you may hear, see, smell, taste or feel things that aren't there. If the areas handling muscle control are overloaded, your muscles may either start contracting violently or completely lose their tone and collapse. If the areas in charge of speech are affected, you may begin babbling incomprehensively or be unable to speak at all. When the electrical currents overload in an area of your brain, you will experience a seizure. And if you have multiple occurrences of such seizures, you have the condition known as epilepsy.

ANATOMY OF AN EPILEPTIC SEIZURE

Epilepsy, also known as *seizure disorder*, is a medical condition characterized by seizures that are brought about by "electrical misfiring" in the brain. This may be the result of a little jolt or a huge flood of electrical current. It might strike in just a small part of the brain or a bigger section, or involve the entire brain.

Excess electrical current is not the only factor that can cause the brain to "seize." Low blood sugar, a very high fever, and other problems can also trigger seizures. This means that not every seizure is an epileptic seizure, and having a seizure does not mean you have epilepsy. Epilepsy is diagnosed only if you have had two or more *unprovoked* seizures; that is, they were not caused by any "outside" factors. But because seizures can arise from many sources, epilepsy can be hard to diagnose. A key issue is determining whether the seizures are epileptic or non-epileptic.

An epileptic seizure originates in the brain, which is made up of trillions of cells called *neurons* which store all of the information we hold in our minds, like memories, ideas, facts, language and so on. The neurons communicate with each other by generating electrical signals that either stimulate (excite) or slow down (inhibit) other neurons. Most of the time, there is a balance between these forces. But when there is either too much excitement or too little inhibition, the excitatory forces dominate and the resulting excess of electrical activity can cause an epileptic seizure.

Depending on how powerful it is and where it strikes, this surge of electricity through the brain can cause a variety of symptoms, ranging from a single, strong muscle contraction to repetitive movements, complete collapse and unconsciousness. Typically, a seizure will last for no longer than a minute or two, although the person may feel confused and exhausted for a much longer period of time.

The Location Determines the Effects

The symptoms of the seizure are directly related to the part of the brain jolted by excess electricity. Since the left half of the brain controls the right side of the body and vice versa; a seizure originating in the brain's left half will affect the right side of the body, while a seizure in the right half of the brain will affect the left side of the body.

But it's not that simple, as each half of the brain is divided in four parts called lobes:

- **The frontal lobe**

Located right behind the forehead, the frontal lobe governs movement, which means that a surge of electricity to one half of the frontal lobe can result in a jerking of the limbs on the opposite side of the body, among other symptoms.

- **The temporal lobe**

Situated close to the ear, the temporal lobe governs auditory sensations, so a surge to this part of the brain might produce auditory hallucinations (voices that no one else could hear), among other symptoms.

- **The parietal lobe**

This lobe, which occupies the top part of the brain, governs bodily sensations, meaning that a surge to the parietal lobe could cause numbness and tingling, among other symptoms.

- **The occipital lobe**

Located at the back of the head, the occipital lobe governs visual sensations, so an "electrical flood" in this area might cause visual hallucinations (visions that no one else could see), among other symptoms.

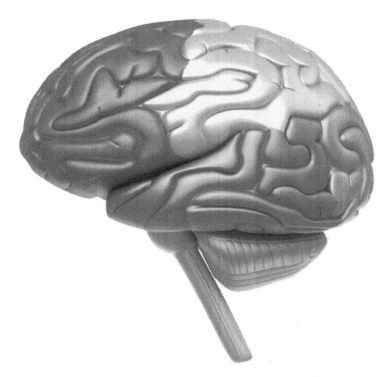

Brain with frontal, temporal, parietal and occipital lobes

Thus, a surge of electricity to the parietal lobe on the left side of the brain might produce numbness and tingling in the right side of the body, while an electrical "jolt" to the frontal lobe on the right side of the brain might produce jerking in the left arm and leg.

Stages of a Seizure

Seizures may occur in three stages, which include an *aura*, the *main seizure*, and the period immediately following the seizure, called the *postical phase*.

Aura

Some people have a feeling or experience certain signs that a seizure is about to happen. These signs, which can include visual disturbances, dizziness, numbness, strange bodily sensations, "butterflies in the stomach," an inability to interact with the outside world and so on, typically occur right before the seizure, last for a few seconds, and could be in occasions remembered very well after the seizure has concluded.

> *Ari, who had simple partial seizures, began experiencing auras at age 21 after one of his friends was killed in a car accident. He described a sensation of déjà vu (feeling like he was repeating a situation that he had never actually experienced), and said there was a funny smell in the air that he could not describe precisely. This experience would last for a few seconds, and would sometimes be followed by a brief staring phase during which he could hear but not respond.*

An aura is the first expression of the seizure, and may occur as an isolated event or an immediate prelude to the main part of the seizure. It's interesting to note that auras only occur in those who have partial epilepsy. (For more information, see "Classifying Epileptic Seizures" later in this chapter.)

Main seizure

A typical seizure can last anywhere from seconds to minutes and take many different forms, from standing still and staring, to violent convulsions and unconsciousness. The characteristics of the seizure may include staring, fluttering of the eyes, lip smacking, lapses of awareness, head drops, loss of posture, sudden collapse, stiffening of the limbs, jerking of the limbs and face, rapid brief contractions of muscles, and unconsciousness, to name a few. The symptoms will depend on the type of seizure and which part of the brain is involved.

Postictal Phase

In most cases, there is a postictal phase (recovery period) after the seizure that lasts from a few seconds to several minutes. In rare cases, it can last for hours or even days. During this time there may be confusion, sleepiness, headaches and occasionally a temporary condition called Todd's paralysis that partially or completely paralyzes one side of the body. The individual may have total recall of the seizure or no memory of it at all.

> *Sharon, a 42 year-old mother of three, had very distinct postictal phases. During her seizures she was unaware of what was happening, and would wake up with a very strong headache, confused and unable to remember how or why she had arrived at that location. It would usually take an hour before Sharon could function normally, and she would continue to have difficulty concentrating for several hours or even a few days. She estimated that it usually took about a week before she felt normal again.*

Most of the time, seizures conclude after several seconds to few minutes without any intervention other than basic first aid. But on rare occasions, they may not stop by themselves. If a seizure continues and become very prolonged, or one seizure immediately follows another (a condition known as *status epilepticus*), the situation may become very dangerous and requires immediate medical care. (See section on "Seizure-Related Emergencies" in Chapter 12 – Practical Issues.)

Epilepsy Myths

Unfortunately, many of the myths that have surrounded epilepsy for centuries are still with us today. These myths, which should forever be put to rest, include:

- *An epileptic seizure is a sign that the person is possessed by the devil.*

- *A person having a seizure is talking to the gods.*

- *People with epilepsy take special medication these days, so they never have seizures.*

- People with epilepsy shouldn't work because it's too stressful.

- Epilepsy is a mental illness.

- People with epilepsy are unable to learn.

- People with epilepsy are aggressive.

- Epilepsy is contagious

- People with epilepsy shouldn't marry and have children.

- If someone is having a seizure, you should put a spoon in their mouth so they won't swallow their tongue.

You can confidently tell anyone and everyone that all of these have *no* basis in fact and are complete and utter myths!

CLASSIFYING EPILEPTIC SEIZURES

Once your doctor has confirmed that your seizures are due to epilepsy, he or she will need to zero in on the type you're experiencing. There are many types of seizures, and you may be affected by more than one. Figuring out which type(s) of seizures you're experiencing is crucial, as it helps determine which medicine(s) are best for you, as well as what you can expect going forward. It may also help clarify the location of the origin of your seizures in your brain.

The classification of epileptic seizures is complex and explicit. To begin with, seizures are divided into two main types: *generalized-onset seizures*, in which the entire brain is affected at once, and *partial-onset seizures*, in which the seizure starts in a specific part of the brain. There are also *secondary generalized seizures,* which begin as partial-onset and then spread, affecting the entire brain, and *infantile spasms* (a special type of seizure), which occur only in very young children. Let's take a quick look at these types.

Generalized-Onset Seizures

In generalized-onset seizures, both sides of the brain are involved from the beginning to the end of the seizure, and a loss of consciousness is experienced with most of them. This category includes absence, atonic, tonic, myoclonic, clonic and tonic-clonic seizures.

Absence seizures

Formerly known as "petit mal" seizures, absence seizures are characterized by brief periods of impaired consciousness (usually less than 20 seconds) that begin and end suddenly. The individual typically stares off into space as if daydreaming and may blink repeatedly, but rarely exhibits other repetitive behavior. After the seizure, the individual returns to normal immediately.

Absence seizures can be brought on by hyperventilation and, in some cases, flashing lights. Commonly attributed to attention deficit disorder (ADD), these seizures most often affect children, but are also seen in some adults and tend to run in families.

> *Michael, a third grader, had difficulty paying attention at school that was mistakenly diagnosed as ADD. His attention problems were actually due to absence seizures, during which he would interrupt what he was doing to stare off into the distance. Because his absence seizures occurred 10 to 20 times per day, they had a definite negative impact on Michael's school performance.*

If the absence seizure lasts longer than a minute or two and the person is confused afterwards, it could represent an *atypical absence seizure*. These are seen mainly in patients with Lennox-Gastaut syndrome, a form of severe childhood-onset epilepsy that usually appears between the ages of 2 and 6.

Atonic seizures

"Atonic" means loss of muscle tone, and these seizures are characterized by a sudden loss of muscle strength that can cause drooping eyelids, a nodding head, the dropping of objects, and falling to the ground ("drop attacks"). The seizures are brief and sudden, and there's a real danger of sustaining head injury. The use of helmets and/or knee pads may be recommended for those who have atonic seizures.

> *Twenty-five year-old Steven had been having seizures since he was 3 months old. But his parents were most concerned about his atonic seizures, the kind that would cause him to lose muscle tone and suddenly fall flat on the ground. To avoid injuries, Steven had to wear a helmet most of the time. He also experienced head drops that lasted for a second, and sometimes occurred in clusters that continued for up to 30 minutes.*

Tonic seizures

Tonic seizures produce symptoms that are the opposite of those seen in atonic seizures. Instead of losing muscle tone, the individual's limbs and/or trunk become stiff. These seizures are brief and sudden and seen mainly in those with Lennox-Gastaut syndrome.

> *Cindy, a cheerful 9 year-old, suffered from tonic seizures during which she would suddenly stiffen both arms, stop breathing, turn blue and fall over. These episodes, which typically lasted between 10 to 20 seconds, sometimes occurred in clusters. Her parents began insisting that she wear a helmet since she had fallen and hit her head several times. Cindy was diagnosed with Lennox-Gastaut syndrome.*

Myoclonic seizures

These seizures are rapid, brief (less than a second) and involve a sudden jerking of the muscles, mostly in the arms and trunk. Myoclonic seizures can occur singly, or in clusters that typically last for a seconds to minutes. (Rest assured that not all jerking episodes are related to epilepsy. Those that occur while drifting off to sleep are generally not due to epilepsy.) People who have myoclonic seizures are often sensitive to strobe lights.

> *Trista started having episodes of hand jerking at the age of 10, mainly in the morning when she first woke up or when she felt tired. Sometimes she would drop the cup or glass she was holding. Her parents took her to a doctor who said that the episodes were due to nervousness, but in fact they were due to juvenile myoclonic epilepsy.*

Clonic seizures

Clonic seizures involve a sudden rhythmic jerking that is similar to that seen in myoclonic seizures, but slower. These seizures are rare and mainly seen in children.

Tonic-clonic seizures

Formerly known as "grand mal" seizures, these are the kind that are most familiar to the general public. They have two phases, *tonic* and *clonic*. During the tonic phase, the individual suddenly becomes stiff, yells loudly, falls to the ground and may have difficulty breathing. During the clonic phase, there is muscle jerking throughout the body. There is always loss of consciousness. Tongue biting and a loss of bladder or bowel control may occur. The seizure lasts from several seconds to a few minutes. After these seizures, the person is usually very tired and confused.

> *There were three signs that would tell 15 year-old Tom that he'd had a tonic-clonic seizure: his body was hurting, he'd wet himself and sometimes his tongue was sore where he had bitten it. He'd wake up with a splitting headache, no memory of what had happened or where he was, and in need of others to tell him what they had witnessed. On more than one occasion, Tom woke up in an emergency room.*

Partial-Onset Seizures

In partial-onset seizures, only a part of the brain is affected by an overload of electrical activity. These seizures can be broken down into two categories: *simple partial*, which do not impair consciousness, and *complex partial*, which do involve a loss of consciousness.

Simple partial seizures

In simple partial seizures, the person is aware and conscious throughout the seizure. It may begin with an aura. Then, depending on the area of the brain involved, there can be jerking or stiffening of certain parts of the body, numbness or tingling, auditory or visual hallucinations, and/or the sensation of smelling something that isn't really there. There may be a feeling of "butterflies in the stomach," sweating and palpitations. A sudden rush of feelings, such as fear, anger, rage, joy or happiness, can occur. There may also be "psychic" feelings, such as déjà vu (a feeling of having experienced a situation that is actually new) or jamais vu (a feeling that a known situation or person is new and unfamiliar).

Complex partial seizures

During a complex partial seizure, the person is not aware of what's happening and afterward will have no memory of the event. Staring and automatic behaviors (such as picking at the clothes or tapping) are the most common manifestations. These seizures can last for several seconds to a few minutes and afterward, the individual is confused.

Secondary Generalized Seizures

This kind of seizure starts in one area of the brain as a simple or complex partial seizure, then evolves into a tonic-clonic seizure that involves the entire brain. The simple partial seizure may first make a "pit stop," becoming a complex partial seizure, but eventually turns into a generalized tonic-clonic seizure. What's important to remember is the seizure begins in one part of the brain but eventually takes over the brain as a whole.

Jim, age 38, had his first seizure when he was 11 months old, while in a feverish state. He then remained seizure free until age 34 when he began to experience episodes of staring off into space, repeating words over and over, smacking his lips and making automatic movements with his hands. In spite of taking high doses of medication, Jim continued to have these seizures, which then turn into generalized tonic-clonic "grand mal" seizures.

Infantile Spasms

These brief episodes of sudden bending forward of the body with stiffening of the arms and legs, or arching back and extending arms and legs occur in very young children, usually between the ages of 3 months and 12 months, and are due to a type of epilepsy called West syndrome. It is very important to diagnose this condition quickly and correctly because if not treated properly, it can result in mental impairment and intractable seizures (seizures that are impossible to control). Diagnosis is based on specific pattern seen on EEG testing called "hypsarrhythmia". A more extensive description of West syndomre (also called "infantile spasms") can be found in chapter 4.

WHAT'S *NOT* AN EPILEPTIC SEIZURE?

Epileptic seizures are caused by an increase in electrical activity in the brain that is non-provoked, which means there is no obvious and immediate reason for the problem. *Non-epileptic seizures* are just the opposite. They are *not* due to electrical surges in the brain and they *are* provoked by physiological or psychological problems or situations. Yet their characteristics are often very similar to epileptic seizures, which can make it hard to differentiate between the two.

Non-epileptic seizures, which can occur singly or in multiples, can be either *physiologic* or *psychological*.

Physiologic Non-Epileptic Seizures

These are "organic" seizures, meaning they originate within the body but are not caused by epilepsy. They may be due to:

- **Fainting** – When a person faints, there is a decrease in blood flow to the brain. If the brain is deprived of oxygen long enough, a seizure could result. Fainting can be caused by various heart conditions such as irregular heartbeat or a vasovagal episode (sudden loss of blood flow to the brain due to changes in the size of the arteries).

- **Low blood sugar (hypoglycemia)** – If the blood sugar level falls too low, convulsions (a type of seizure) may follow. These are seen most often in patients with diabetes who are taking medications to lower the blood sugar, and those who experience frequent changes in blood sugar levels.

- **Changes in electrolyte levels (i.e. sodium, calcium, magnesium and potassium)** – Electrolytes are substances with the capacity to conduct electricity, and when their levels are abnormal, they affect the electrical activity of the brain and can produce seizures. Electrolyte balance may be disrupted by dehydration, severe vomiting, laxative abuse and other problems. Even some of antiseizure medications can lower sodium levels, such as carbamazepine (Tegretol®) or oxcarbazepine (Trileptal®). This can, although infrequently, also trigger this type of non-epileptic seizures.

- **Toxins** – Various prescribed medications, chemotherapy, alcohol and illicit drugs have all been associated with seizures.

- **Fever** – Seizures (known as febrile seizures) sometimes occur in response to a high fever, typically in children between the ages of 6 months and 5 years.

None of the above constitutes epilepsy.

Psychological Non-Epileptic Seizures (PNES)

Stress or other psychological conditions can sometimes trigger psychological non-epileptic seizures (PNES). These seizures are treated with psychotherapy and, when necessary, psychiatric medication. The situation becomes more confusing when patients suffer from both epileptic and PNES seizures.

It May Look Like An Epileptic Seizure, But It Isn't...

Many conditions can produce seizures or other symptoms that might be mistaken for epilepsy. They include:

- **Stroke and transient ischemic attacks (TIAs)** - Strokes and TIAs result from a significant drop in blood flow to the brain which causes the death of brain cells. If the stroke is brief, it could be mistaken for a seizure.

- **Migraine headaches** - Sometimes migraines are accompanied by neurological disturbances such as changes in vision, weakness, speech difficulties or numbness, all of which can be also symptoms of seizures.

- **Movement disorders** - Tic disorders (uncontrolled movement), temporary violent movements like chorea, and temporary tremors are often mistaken for seizures.

- **Sleep disorders** - Sleep talking, sleep walking and jerking movements while falling asleep are sometimes mistaken for seizures. In addition, "REM behavior disorder", in which an individual acts out dreams, can cause what looks like being awake in the middle of the night and staring, looking confused, moving from place to place, or automatic behavior. This behavior can be mistaken for complex partial seizures

- **Anxiety/panic disorder** - Panic attacks can be confused with partial seizures associated with intense fear.

- **Vertigo** - These episodes of dizziness are sometimes mistaken for simple partial seizures, which can have vertigo as a symptom.

- **Cardiac disorders** - Changes in heart rhythm can lead to decreased blood flow and fainting. Both of these might be mistaken for epilepsy, as they can result in seizures when prolonged enough.

- **Episodic dyscontrol syndrome (rage attacks)** - This is a pattern of unprovoked outbursts of frequently violent and uncontrollable social behavior. This syndrome can be mistaken for complex partial seizures.

- **Breath-holding spells** - Children who have tantrums and cry for prolonged periods of time may hold their breath for several seconds, which can trigger an episode that looks like a seizure.

It's extremely important to distinguish correctly between epileptic and non-epileptic seizures as their treatments are very different, and the consequences of a wrong diagnosis can be devastating. For example, treatments for epileptic seizures can include anticonvulsant medications, diet, implants and even brain surgery, while the treatments for non-epileptic seizures involve completely different medications, possibly including psychiatric medications and psychotherapy.

You can see how harmful it would be to treat a patient who has epileptic seizures with an antidepressant, and a patient who has non-epileptic seizures due to stress with an anticonvulsant or surgery! Yet many patients who have been diagnosed with epilepsy and are taking antiepileptic medication do not actually have epileptic seizures! *In fact, it's estimated that 20 to 30 percent of patients referred to epilepsy centers do not have epilepsy.*

Now that you know that seizures can be epileptic or non-epileptic, you know why it's so important that your doctor completes a thorough medical history, physical exam, appropriate tests and video-EEG monitoring to confirm that your seizures are, in fact, due to epilepsy, not something else. (For more on this, see Chapter 3 – Diagnosing Epilepsy.)

WHAT TYPE OF EPILEPSY DO YOU HAVE?

Once it's been determined that you *do* have epilepsy, and the kind of epileptic seizure you've experienced has been identified, you're two big steps closer to a finding out which type of epilepsy you have. The type of epilepsy is diagnosed by considering two main factors:

- *The type of epileptic seizures* - Are they generalized-onset or partial-onset? Atonic? Myoclonic? Tonic clonic?

- *The cause of the epilepsy* - Is it idiopathic (no known cause) or symptomatic (the cause is known)? If it's symptomatic, what exactly is the cause? Possibilities include head injury, stroke, brain tumors, brain infections, brain malformations, genetic factors, problems during birth and delivery, and others.

By combining both seizure type and the cause, we can not only zero in on the type of epilepsy you have, but also determine the expected progression of the disorder and (most importantly) the correct treatment.

In the next two chapters, we'll take a look at the causes of epilepsy in depth and examine the methods used to arrive at a correct diagnosis.

CHAPTER TWO
WHAT CAUSES IT AND WHO'S AT RISK?

●

What do Julius Caesar, Napoleon Bonaparte, Michelangelo, Vincent van Gogh, singer/composer Neil Young and Agatha Christie have in common? They either had, or are believed to have had, epilepsy. Other famous and accomplished people who belong to this group include Sir Isaac Newton, Charles Dickens, President Theodore Roosevelt, actor Richard Burton and Olympic hockey player Chandra Gunn.

And then, of course, there are the millions of "regular folks" who have epilepsy yet lead productive, happy and fulfilling lives. In the U.S., the likelihood of having epileptic seizures is nearly 1 in 100, which means that some 2.5 million Americans will be affected by epilepsy at some point in their lives. Yet anyone could have a seizure. All it takes is for something to happen that causes an electrical overload in the brain that exceeds what's called the *seizure threshold*.

THE SEIZURE THRESHOLD

The seizure threshold is the amount of stimulus necessary to produce a seizure. It's like the threshold at the entrance to your house, that little piece of metal or wood that sits beneath your door. Once you step over that threshold, you're in the house.

Most people have a naturally high threshold for seizures. This means that it's not easy to produce an electrical overload in their brains, as the physical and chemical structures that control the flow of electrical current are finely tuned. For other people, the threshold is lower, and may be very low. But whether the threshold is naturally high or low, certain factors such as sleep deprivation, stress, fever and traveling through time zones can lower it. This means that even people with high thresholds can suffer a seizure, if situations and/or substances lower it far enough.

To understand how the seizure threshold works, think in terms of numbers and a wall. (The numbers in this example are arbitrary but they make the point.) Imagine the seizure threshold is a wall that protects the brain, and for most people that wall is, let's say, 100 inches tall. As long as the wall is there, excessive amounts of seizure-causing currents cannot get through to the brain. However, that wall can be chipped away by seizure-causing factors.

Let's suppose you're born with some structural variations in your brain that leave you with a slightly lower wall, one that stands only 90 inches tall. You're starting off with a little less protection than average, but it's still sufficient. Then you get very busy with work and family and become sleep deprived. The resulting physical stress knocks about 20 inches off the top of your wall. Then your grandmother dies, and the emotional stress knocks off another 30 inches. At this point, your 90-inch wall is down to just 40 inches. You then develop a fever, which shaves off 20 more inches, and due to a very hot summer you get dehydrated and your electrolytes become unbalanced. This knocks away the remaining 20 inches of your wall. You now have absolutely no protection and wham! You suddenly have a seizure. There was no sole cause of the seizure; many factors contributed.

Although in the previous example we could list the factors that contributed to the seizure, sometimes the threshold is lowered for unknown reasons. As a result, seizures occur more easily and with less provocation. We call these *breakthrough seizures.*

COMMON CAUSES OF EPILEPSY

As scientific knowledge expands and technology improves, we become better able to understand why some people have thresholds low enough to allow epileptic seizures to occur. But about half of the time we simply have no answer.

The cause of epilepsy is labeled *idiopathic* when we don't know why it began, and *symptomatic* when we do know why it began. Idiopathic causes include genetic factors. Symptomatic causes include head injury, stroke, brain tumors, brain infections, brain malformations, metabolic problems like diabetes, problems during pregnancy and delivery, and others.

Any brain can develop epilepsy, but those with the following genetic and non-genetic problems are more susceptible.

Genetic Abnormalities Associated With Epilepsy
Epilepsy frequently has a genetic basis. There are many types of epilepsy that run in families, and literally hundreds of inherited conditions have seizures as a feature. Genetic problems occur either in the chromosomes or the genes.

Every cell in your body contains all of your genetic information in the form of DNA. The DNA is packaged in chromosomes, which you can think of as "books" in a library. Each chromosome is made up of hundreds of genes, which are like the words contained in the book. Each gene, in turn, is made up of a sequence of DNA base-pairs, which are like the letters making up the words in the book. The DNA tells a given cell how to carry out a particular task, such as making a protein.

Chromosomal problems occur when there is either an abnormal number of chromosomes or the structure of a certain chromosome is defective. For example, a defect in chromosome 20 causes it to have an abnormal ring shape and to produce severe epilepsy.

Genetic problems could also result from changes that occur in the DNA sequence, which are called mutations. Mutations change the way the cell works, causing it to create proteins that may work improperly. When these proteins are involved in brain formation or metabolism or communication within the brain, there can be an increase in electrical activity or a lessening of the brain's natural inhibitory factors. Either of these can set off an electrical surge that becomes an epileptic seizure.

- **Mutations of genes involved in brain formation** – While the embryo is forming, the brain cells of an embryo must travel from their place of origin to their permanent location, if the brain is to form properly. Genes tell the cells where to go, but mutations can scramble these instructions. If the brain cells go to the wrong spot, there may be faulty "brain wiring" and the creation of an area in the brain that produces seizures (known as a "seizure focus.") For example, some genetic mutations can cause an abnormality called *lissencephaly,* which means "smooth brain." In this mutation, because the neurons don't migrate properly, the folds that normally occur on the surface of the brain are lacking, resulting in intellectual disabilities, neurological deficits and, frequently, seizures.

- **Mutations of genes involved in brain metabolism** – Genes are responsible for making proteins called enzymes that break down other proteins in the cell. When mutations occur, production of a particular enzyme may decrease, allowing the build-up of corresponding proteins in the brain cells. As protein levels build up, brain cells can become damaged or die, producing seizures. Tay-Sachs disease, for example, occurs when a protein in the brain builds up and causes neurological deterioration. Symptoms begin at about 6 months of age and the child usually dies by the age of 4.

- **Mutations of genes involved in brain communication** Brain cells communicate with each other using electrical impulses, which in turn, are generated by protein structures called ion channels. Ion channels generate electrical charges by carefully controlling the leakage of electrolytes (e.g. sodium) into and out of the brain cells. Mutations in the genes that control the "blueprints" for these ion channels can cause conduction of the wrong amount of electrolytes into the cells. This can result in brain cells that are too excitable or not very good at inhibiting other excitable cells. Patients with these mutations are more likely to suffer from epileptic seizures. Severe myclonic epilepsy of infancy (SMEI), also known Dravet's Syndrome, is linked to this type of mutation.

As with all genetic disorders, inherited epilepsy may affect one family member while sparing others or even skipping several generations. In some cases, such as familial frontal lobe epilepsy, there is a gene that controls this kind of epilepsy and any family member who has that gene will develop the disorder. In other cases, just like we saw with absence epilepsy, there is no obvious genetic marker, yet there is a clear family tendency toward developing the disorder.

Head Injury
Two to 35 percent of those who suffer head injuries will begin having seizures afterwards, a condition referred to as post-traumatic epilepsy. Trauma to the head causes changes in the brain that can lead to bleeding and swelling, which can result in the irritation or death of brain cells and the creation of scar tissue. This scar tissue affects the normal flow of electrical activity in the brain and can lower the seizure threshold. Either partial or generalized seizures can follow.

The development of epilepsy is more likely in cases of severe trauma, open or penetrating wounds, bleeding in the brain, coma that lasts more than a day, and/or seizures that occur soon after the injury. In more than half the cases, seizures develop within a year of the head injury; in 80 percent, they develop within two years. However, some seizures don't begin until ten or more years after the injury.

Stroke

Stroke, the sudden death of brain cells due to a disturbance in the blood supply to the brain, is the most common cause of epilepsy in the elderly, although it can also occur in younger people.

There are two kinds of stroke: *ischemic stroke*, caused by a lack of blood flow to part of the brain, resulting in tissue death in that area; and *hemorrhagic stroke*, damage to the brain due to a ruptured blood vessel that bleeds into the surrounding tissue. Approximately 10 percent of those with ischemic strokes will develop epilepsy, compared to 20 to 30 percent with hemorrhagic strokes. Post-stroke epilepsy is also more likely to occur if the stroke is large or involves the cortex (outer part of the brain).

Brain Tumors

Between 30 and 50 percent of those who have brain tumors will develop seizures and epilepsy. Large tumors and those that are located in the frontal and parietal lobes or the cortex, are more likely to cause epilepsy. The tumor types most likely to be associated with seizures and epilepsy include:

- **Metastases** – A secondary tumor that has spread from the original tumor to the brain. One of the most common examples of this is the skin cancer known as melanoma.

- **Dysembryoplastic neuroepithelial tumor (DNET)** – A type of brain tumor, particularly in young people that can cause epilepsy with long-standing drug-resistant partial seizures.

- **Ganglioglioma** – A type of central nervous system tumor that frequently occurs in the temporal lobe of the brain and can cause epilepsy.

- **Gliobastoma multiforme (GBM)** – A malignant brain tumor typically associated with neuropsychological decline, seizures and ultimately death.

- **Meningioma** – A type of benign tumor that grows from the lining of the brain (meninges). These tumors are typically slow growing but can cause problems by compressing the brain or spinal cord.

- **Low-grade astrocytoma** – This slow-growing tumor, which arises from a brain cell called an astrocyte, can cause seizures and has the potential to progress to higher grade tumors such as GBMs.

Brain Infections

Epilepsy can be caused by infections of the brain itself (encephalitis) or the covering of the brain (meningitis). These infections can be caused by many things including viruses (e.g. herpes), bacteria (e.g. meningococcus, pneumococcus), fungi or parasites. The risk of developing epilepsy is higher with encephalitis and more difficult to control. It may have more than one point of origin, making it impossible to treat surgically.

Brain Malformations

As I mentioned above in the section on Genetic Abnormalities, when an embryo is forming in the uterus, the brain cells (neurons) must travel a certain pathway to reach their final destination in the brain. In those with migrational disorders, the neurons travel to the wrong place or stop before reaching their proper destination, resulting in structurally abnormal cerebral hemispheres. The brain malformations, with names like *polymicrogyria, macrogyria, schizencephaly* and *cortical dysplasia,* can range from mild to severe. If they are located in a single part of the brain, it may be possible to surgically remove them.

Metabolic Disorders

Certain endocrine disorders may be associated with seizures and epilepsy (sometimes can provoke physiological non epileptic seizures and in other occasions can be the cause of epilepsy), including:

- **Diabetes/hypoglycemia** – Diabetes is a disease of excessive glucose (sugar) in the blood, while hypoglycemia is the opposite – too little blood glucose. Some with diabetes can experience both conditions when treatments drive blood glucose levels too low, producing hypoglycemia. Either state can produce seizures, as both are brain irritants that may cause irreversible brain injury. Seizures can compound this injury.

- **Thyroid dysfunction** – Severe hyperthyroidism (high-functioning thyroid) causes excessive metabolic activity in multiple organs, including the brain. When extreme metabolic demands are placed on the brain cells, seizures can result. Milder hyperthyroidism and hypothyroidism (low-functioning thyroid) have also been reported to worsen seizure control, but there is no definitive proof of this.

- **Parathyroid disorders** – If your parathyroid glands make too little parathyroid hormone (PTH), your blood will have abnormally low levels of calcium, an electrolyte that helps make brain cells less excitable. Too little PTH, therefore, can make brain cells more excitable and prone to seizures.

- **Adrenal insufficiency** – In this condition, the adrenal glands do not produce enough aldosterone, which regulates blood levels of sodium and potassium. When levels of these important electrolytes are imbalanced, seizures can result. Adrenal insufficiency or failure can also cause the kidneys to fail, producing a build-up of toxins in the blood that can irritate brain cells and cause seizures.

Degenerative Diseases

People with Alzheimer's disease have a higher chance of developing seizures.

Perinatal Factors

The developing brain of the fetus and baby is very susceptible to damage. If the mother-to-be contracts an infection, takes certain substances, eats poorly or lacks oxygen, the baby's brain could sustain damage, resulting in epileptic seizures. Complications during delivery and first weeks of life can also result in lack of oxygen or other types of injuries to developing brain, resulting in epilepsy.

Other Less Common Causes

There are also many less common causes of epilepsy, including the following:

- **Cardiac disorders** – These may affect blood flow to the brain, causing a stroke that increases the risk of seizures.

- **Gastrointestinal and liver conditions** – Various gastrointestinal and liver conditions can affect the absorption and use of medications, increasing the risk of seizures. Additionally, some experts speculate that seizures and gastrointestinal absorption problems share a common autoimmune mechanism, causing the immune system to attack both the brain and the gastrointestinal cells.

- **Blood problems** – Diseases in which the blood is abnormally prone to clotting (such as sickle cell disease) can result in strokes due to a blockage of blood flow to the brain. Those with the opposite condition, hemophilia, have trouble forming clots, which can produce strokes due to brain hemorrhage. Either way, a stroke can produce brain damage that causes seizures.

- **Inflammatory diseases** – Lupus, Sjogren's syndrome, Crohn's disease and other diseases with an inflammatory component can produce seizures.

- **Multiple sclerosis, sarcoidosis and vasculitis** – Those who have these diseases may suffer seizures as a result of strokes or autoimmune damage to the brain cells.

- **Organ transplants** – Epilepsy can result from associated infections or the medications used in transplantations.

- **Poisons** – Lead poisoning can produce severe neurologic injury and seizures, but the exposure to lead must be unusually high. Those who eat shellfish containing high amounts of demoic acid (produced by toxic algae blooms that have been consumed by the animal) can develop seizures as well as short term memory loss. Demoic acid activates proteins in the memory center of the brain that cause an excessive influx of calcium, causing cell death.

- **Respiratory problems** – Severe sleep apnea and respiratory insufficiency cause a decrease in brain oxygenation that can irritate brain cells and produce seizures.

- **Kidney problems** – Diseased kidneys are ineffective at removing toxins from the bloodstream, so toxin levels rise, brain cells may become irritated, and a seizure can result. Brain cell irritation and seizures can also occur when kidney dialysis (filtering of the blood through a machine) causes sudden changes in the blood's electrolyte balance.

Of course, not everyone who has an alteration in brain formation, develops an infection, or has another factor that increases susceptibility will go on to develop epilepsy. Such people are certainly more at risk, but there must be something that "pushes them over the edge" before seizures can occur. We call that something a trigger.

SEIZURE TRIGGERS

Seizure triggers are environmental or personal factors that can bring on seizures but do not, by themselves, cause seizures. A trigger is that last blow that lowers the seizure threshold "wall" enough to allow an electrical brainstorm. Many people with epilepsy have seizure triggers, the most common being sleep deprivation, alcohol withdrawal, recreational drugs, hyperventilation, emotional stress, environmental temperature changes, exposure to flickering lights, fever or illness, hormonal changes, medications and supplements, missed medications, time of day and traveling across time zones.

It's very important that you discover your own seizure triggers. I strongly suggest that you keep a journal or a seizure calendar to document when and where your seizures took place and all of the factors that might have contributed (e.g. too little sleep, the menstrual cycle, stress, exhaustive exercise, illness, and so on). Once you know what may be triggering your seizures, you can take steps to minimize or eliminate those factors and achieve better seizure control.

Now let's take a closer look at the triggers most likely to bring about a seizure.

Alcohol and Recreational Drugs

Alcohol can precipitate seizures not by its use, but by its withdrawal. Alcohol raises the seizure threshold by making the brain cells less excitable, but when the blood alcohol level suddenly decreases, the brain cells become hyperexcitable. Thus, when people drink large amounts of alcohol there is an increased chance of "day after" seizures. Long-term use/abuse of alcohol also causes a deficiency of important vitamins and other nutrients that could lead to seizures.

The recreational drugs associated with seizures are mainly cocaine and amphetamines. These drugs generate an excessive release of excitatory neurotransmitters that can trigger seizures. Cocaine can also cause a narrowing of the blood vessels (vasculitis) and strokes. Additionally, those who indulge in recreational drugs are more likely to fall and sustain injuries to the head or brain, which can cause seizures. For all of these reasons, anyone prone to seizures should abstain from using alcohol and recreational drugs.

Emotional Stress

Stress can trigger seizures by causing insomnia and sleep deprivation, or anxiety-provoked hyperventilation. It may also favor seizures for reasons yet to be discovered. At any rate, it is a strong trigger for epileptic seizures and should be controlled. While simply avoiding stress would be ideal, life doesn't work that way. However, practicing relaxation techniques such as yoga and meditation, taking short breaks and getting a massage are all good ways to reduce and relieve stress. If stress becomes unmanageable, therapy is an option you should discuss with your doctor.

Environmental Temperature Changes

Sudden changes in temperature, as in going from any icy, air-conditioned room into the hot sun, can lead to seizures in those with Dravet syndrome (severe myoclonic epilepsy in infancy). It is unknown why this rare type of epilepsy is sensitive to temperature changes.

Exposure to Flickering Lights

This kind of trigger is more common in those who have myoclonic (jerking) seizures. People with photosensitivity may be sensitive to different visual patterns, including flashing lights, strobe lights, video games, TV waves, or even sunlight flickering through leaves on a bright day, creating a strobe-like affect. While avoidance of these visual patterns is ideal, it's not always possible. Using non-glare glasses, polarized sunglasses, flicker-free computer monitors and monitor glare guards can be helpful. Also, when working on the computer, it's a good idea to take frequent breaks and stay not too close to the screen.

Fever or Illness

The presence of fever, colds or any illness can lower the seizure threshold and allow initial or breakthrough seizures. The doctor should always be informed when sickness occurs, especially if there is vomiting and the possibility of not holding on to medications, so proper treatment can be administered.

Hormonal Changes

Changes in hormones can have significant effects on seizures. In males, puberty and changes in hormones can play a role in epilepsy. In females, seizures may be related to a certain time in menstrual cycle. This is referred to as "catamenial epilepsy." Seizures can also get better or worse during pregnancy and menopause, when the female body undergoes significant changes in hormonal levels. (For more on this, see "Women's Issues" in Chapter 10 – Special Medical Concerns; and Chapter 11 – Pregnancy – Before, During and After).

Hyperventilation

Hyperventilating (over-breathing) is another potent factor that could trigger seizures. This occurs especially in absence seizures. Those with hyperventilation as a trigger should avoid exhaustive exercise. It may be possible to play sports, as long as they don't involve extreme physical exertion. (For more on this, see the section on "Exercise and Sports" in Chapter 12 – Practical Issues.)

Sleep Deprivation

Sleep deprivation is one of the most potent triggers for seizures. This is commonly seen in adolescents and young adults who stay up late to study, socialize or avoid going to bed. No one knows exactly why a lack of sleep can trigger seizures. And while there is no set number of hours of sleep that any one person needs (some need 6 hours, others 10), most people know how much they need to feel refreshed. When going to bed late is unavoidable, getting extra sleep the next morning is advised. (For more on this, see "Epilepsy and Sleep" in Chapter 10 – Special Medical Concerns.)

Time of Day

Seizures that occur mainly during sleep are called "nocturnal seizures." "Diurnal seizures" occur during the day when the person is awake. And there are others that occur at either time. If seizures occur at a specific time of day, the doctor may adjust the timing of the medication to afford more protection. However, the pattern could change over time and further adjustments may be needed.

Medications and Supplements

Numerous medications (prescription and over-the-counter), as well as herbal supplements, can potentially make seizures worse. You can find a list of the medications that could provoke seizures in Appendix 4.

Missed Medications

The importance of taking medication as prescribed cannot be stressed strongly enough.

Non-compliance with medications is one of the most frequent and significant triggers of breakthrough seizures. We see this in those who shun medications because they are "unnatural" and cause side effects. Adolescents often miss doses because they think they don't need medications or they forget to take them. Patients with memory problems, which is very common in epilepsy, may forget to take medication. Becoming better educated about the risks of missing doses may help those who resist medication. Those with memory problems might benefit from using pill organizers or other strategies to remind them to take medications.

Traveling Across Time Zones

When travelling across time zones, sleep deprivation is almost inevitable and the times that medications are taken will change. It's a good idea to catch up on sleep the first night and to take two clocks: one set for local time and the other for the time it is at home. Medication should always be taken according to the home clock.

PREVENTING SEIZURES BY CONTROLLING TRIGGERS

While not every epileptic seizure can be avoided, you can do much to prevent them by doing the following:

- Use a journal or seizure calendar to document your seizures and all possible contributing factors (e.g. too little sleep, menstrual cycle, stress, exhaustive exercise, illness and so on).

- Once you are aware of your triggers, take steps to control or avoid them.

- Avoid alcohol and recreational drugs.

- Refrain from exhaustive exercise if hyperventilation is a trigger for you.

- Learn to defuse, control and release emotional stress.

- Be careful of environmental temperature changes. Wear clothing in layers so it can be removed or added as needed.

- Avoid exposure to flickering lights. Use non-glare glasses, polarized sunglasses, flicker-free computer monitors and monitor glare guards.

- See your doctor immediately if you develop a fever or any serious illness.

- Consult your doctor for advice regarding hormonal changes.

- Avoid medications and supplements that are known seizure triggers. Mention all medications or supplements you are taking to your doctor

- Take your anti-epileptic medications exactly as prescribed. Use pill organizers and other strategies to help you remember.

- Get plenty of sleep.

- Get extra sleep when traveling across time zones.

- If you experience seizures at a particular time of day, talk to your doctor about adjusting the timing of your medication.

- If you are afraid of taking a certain medication or medications in general, or you are experiencing uncomfortable side effects, talk to your doctor immediately. He or she should be able to come up with an acceptable solution.

Understanding your triggers can help you control your seizures. Some triggers, like time of day, can indicate when your medication will be most effective. Others, like missed medication, alcohol or seizure-inducing medications, can be prevented. Still others, like sleep deprivation, stress and flickering lights can usually be minimized, if not avoided.

My 11 year-old patient, Gina, is a good example of someone whose seizure control involves trigger avoidance. Gina started having seizures at age 2, mostly while riding in the car on sunny days. Her eyes would flutter and roll back in her head, but she remained alert during the episodes. Her mother started putting a hat on her whenever she went out in the sunlight. One day, at age 7, Gina was outdoors on a swing without her hat and suddenly fell and started jerking. Her pediatric neurologists ran an EEG and confirmed photosensitivity. They treated her with Keppra®, which didn't help, and Depakote®, which was discontinued because it caused significant weight gain.

When Gina came to me she was on Lamictal® and still experiencing uncontrollable seizures. While taking down her family history, I learned that her father had a similar type of epilepsy. I admitted her for video-EEG monitoring and confirmed a diagnosis of photosensitive generalized epilepsy with absence and myoclonic seizures. Depakote® was tried again, this time with a calorie-controlled diet to prevent weight gain plus strong measures to prevent photosensitivity (using a hat all times, wearing polarized sunglasses). I'm happy to say that Gina has been seizure free now for several months.

The more you know about your seizures and what's bringing them on, the more power you have to control them and keep seizures at bay. Learn all you can!

CHAPTER THREE
DIAGNOSING EPILEPSY

When I first met Marnie, she was 7 years old with uncontrolled seizures that significantly affected her quality of life. Her seizures mainly consisted of sudden bouts of staring (not preceded by an aura) that lasted 10 to 40 seconds and occurred up to 100 times a day. Marnie's former doctors had tried multiple anticonvulsants with no success and she was diagnosed with intractable (untreatable) absence epilepsy. Although she had superior intelligence, she was having difficulty in school due to the constant interruptions, and the powerful medications she was taking fatigued her.

I performed general and neurological exams on Marnie, followed by a video-EEG, which showed evidence of left frontal involvement. It soon became clear that even though her seizures "looked" like absence seizures, they were actually complex partial seizures of left frontal onset. A pre-surgical evaluation showed that a left frontal lobectomy was indicated. Marnie had the surgery and improved significantly, as did her school performance. Today, at age 20, Marnie very rarely experiences a seizure and takes minimal medication.

It's crucial that your doctor correctly diagnose and classify your particular type of epilepsy in order to determine the most effective treatments. The right diagnosis will narrow the choice of medications, as some types will respond well to certain groups of medication but get worse with others. It can also determine whether or not surgery is an option. Surgery may be warranted in some cases, but in others it may do nothing at all or even make things worse. And it can answer important questions about the progression of the disorder: Will it recede over time? Perhaps disappear completely? Or continue indefinitely? The process begins with the collection of information from many sources, including various tests.

COLLECTING INFORMATION AND TESTING

Your doctor will diagnose and classify your epilepsy by analyzing information obtained from your medical history, physical examination, blood tests, a routine or prolonged EEG and possibly a CT scan, MRI or other imaging study. Let's take a look at each of these diagnostic steps.

Medical History

Diagnosis and classification of your epilepsy type begins with a thorough medical history. You will be the primary source for the history, but interviews with your family members or friends can also provide valuable information, especially regarding seizures that you may not remember well, if at all. Your doctor will ask you important questions like:

- When did you have your first seizure?

- How frequent are the seizures?

- Do you remember the seizures?

- Are the seizures preceded by an aura?

- What do the seizures look like?

- How long do they last?

- What happens after the seizures? For example, are you sleepy? Confused? Is it hard to talk?

- How long does it take to get back to normal?

- Are you aware of anything that may trigger the seizures?

- Do you have a family history of epilepsy?

- What kind of testing has been done already?

- Are there any associated medical conditions such as lupus or kidney problems?

- Have you been treated previously? If so, which treatments (medications, diets, surgeries) have been used?

- Are you allergic to any medications? If so, which ones?

Before your appointment, it will be very helpful if you make notes about your medical history, think about your answers to the questions listed above and try to remember anything else that may be related to your seizures. Then take these notes with you to your appointment.

Physical Exam

You may wonder what a physical examination can reveal: after all, epilepsy occurs in the brain, not the body. But the physical exam can sometimes help identify the cause of the epilepsy. Examination of the skin, for example, might reveal characteristics of some skin conditions related to seizures, such as tuberous sclerosis or Sturge-Weber disease.

Observing you physically may also help identify the type of epilepsy. For example, absence epilepsy seizures can be provoked by hyperventilation, so your doctor may ask you to hyperventilate to see if this might trigger an episode.

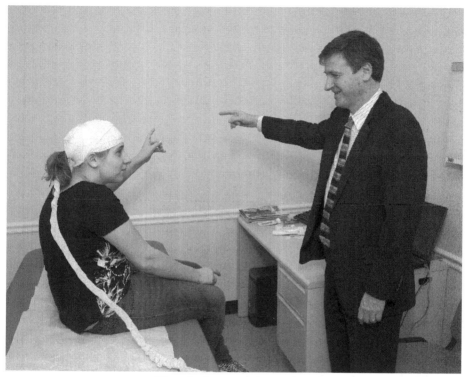

Neurologist examining patient

Tests

Even if your medical history and a physical examination provide a wealth of information, it should be supplemented and possibly verified by testing. These tests will probably include blood work and a routine EEG, and may include some form of imaging (such as a CT scan or MRI) and a prolonged EEG.

- **Test - Checking the Blood**

Analysis of the blood can be very helpful in pinpointing a diagnosis. It may reveal important clues such as electrolyte imbalances (low sodium or calcium levels, changes in potassium levels), kidney or liver problems, hormonal abnormalities (diabetes or thyroid problems) and various metabolic problems including phenylketonuria (PKU). Blood work may also help rule *out* epilepsy by identifying hypoglycemia or other factors that could be causing non-epileptic seizures.

- **Test - Routine EEG**

The EEG (electroencephalogram) measures electrical activity in the brain, just as the EKG (electrocardiogram) monitors the electrical activity of the heart. The EEG is used to establish that you are truly having epileptic seizures. (While it's possible that you *appear* to be having an epileptic seizure, if your brain shows no seizure activity, it will be classified as a "nonepileptic event.") For example, a seizure experienced by a child running a high fever is not considered epilepsy.

How it's done

For an EEG, numerous electrodes are placed on the scalp to detect electrical activity in the brain. This information is transmitted to the EEG machine, which produces a series of wavy lines representing electrical activity in different areas of the brain, much like the recording of tremors during an earthquake by a seismograph. A routine EEG, which usually lasts between 20 to 60 minutes, can be performed while the patient is awake, drowsy or asleep. Sometimes the doctor will try to trigger epileptic activity using provocative measures such as exposure to flashing lights, sleep deprivation, or induced hyperventilation. The goal is to try to "catch" the changes in the brain's electrical activity during a seizure and register them on the graph. However, the activity registered between seizures is also of a lot of value.

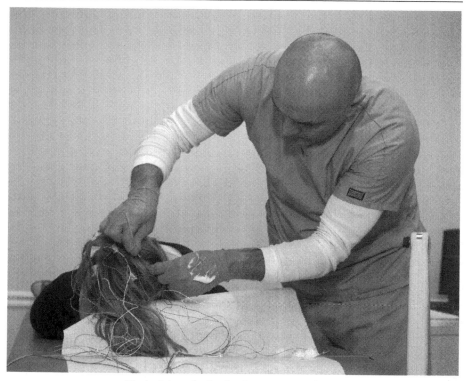

Technician placing leads on patient's head

What it shows

In those who do *not* have epilepsy, all of the wavy lines will show balanced activity, which is represented by "calm" wave patterns. But in those who do have epilepsy, some of the lines (in partial epilepsy) or all of them (in generalized epilepsy) will have "spikes" indicating excessive electrical activity. These spikes, which look like sharp points on the graph, suggest (but don't prove) that there is a tendency (more chances) to have seizures.

Spikes are considered suggestive of a seizure disorder because they can occur even when a seizure is not in progress – although there will be typical activity that is much more evident during a seizure. When spikes occur even when the patient is not having a seizure, those areas of the brain are assumed to be more excitable and, therefore, more seizure-prone.

During a seizure, most of the time we see rhythmic activity that represents the firing of many brain cells at the same time, instead of spikes. The location of this activity may be so well-defined it can indicate the exact place of seizure origin in the brain. Or there may be no spikes or rhythmic activity at all, because the affected area is so small it doesn't produce enough electrical activity to be picked up by a routine EEG. In this case, a prolonged EEG might be the next step. (See section on the Prolonged EEG below.)

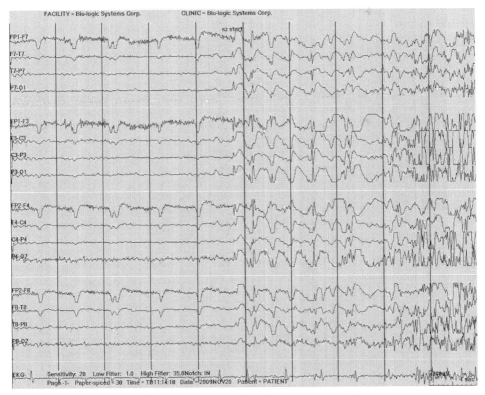

Normal EEG on left and epileptiform activity on the right

It's Not Just a Matter of Spikes

It's important to note that not all patients with EEG spikes have epilepsy. About 2% of the non-epileptic population have EEG spikes and *never* develop seizures or epilepsy. Thus, an "abnormal" EEG by itself does *not* confirm the diagnosis of epilepsy. On the other hand, it is possible for a patient who does have epilepsy to produce an EEG without spikes. Thus, a "normal" EEG does not conclusively rule out epilepsy.

- **Test - Prolonged EEG**

When a routine EEG doesn't clarify the diagnosis sufficiently, a prolonged EEG, which could last anywhere from a few hours to several days, may be required. Most of the prolonged EEG devices have an "event button" for you to press every time you think a seizure (or anything else unusual) is about to occur. Your doctor can see on the EEG when you pushed the event button and will scrutinize those parts of the test very carefully.

Prolonged EEGs may be performed in the hospital and require the tapering off any anti-epileptic medications with the goal of capturing a seizure in progress. Or they may be done at home (an ambulatory EEG).

When it's used

Prolonged EEGs are used:

o when epilepsy is suspected

o to differentiate between epileptic and non-epileptic events

o to determine the specific type of epilepsy

o when the patient is not responding to treatment

o when epilepsy surgery is being considered

Video-EEG

The most common type of prolonged EEG is the video-EEG, which combines videotape monitoring with recording of an EEG. Mostly conducted in a safe hospital environment, the video EEG is considered the best way to understand a patient's epilepsy and locate the "seizure focus," or the part of the brain where the seizure originates.

Since the objective is to catch a seizure in progress, your doctor may decrease any anti-seizure medications you may be taking and might also use seizure-inducing techniques such as sleep deprivation, induced hyperventilation and strobe light stimulation (always in the hospital in a safe environment). If and when a seizure does occur, your doctor will be able to observe your seizure behaviors on the video and interpret your EEG waves. An in-hospital video-EEG test may require a stay of up to several days.

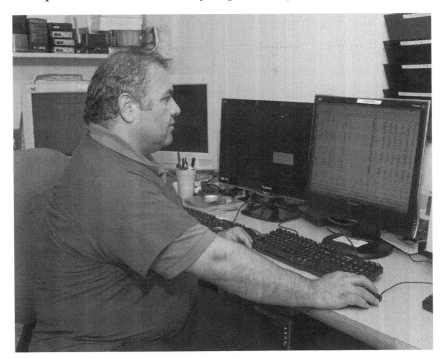

Technician preparing EEG information for the epilepsy specialist

Ambulatory EEG

The advantage of an ambulatory EEG is that no hospitalization is required and you may be able to go about your routine activities. The disadvantage is that your anti-seizure medications cannot be decreased for this test (since you're not in a hospital environment), so there may be no seizure to monitor. Also, if the equipment fails, the entire study can be lost since there is no way to detect a mechanical problem until the recorder is returned to the doctor.

Test – More sophisticated type of brain activity recording

Magnetoencephalogram (MEG)

MEG is a technique that records magnetic fields associated with electrical activity in brain. Electrical activity is also recorded by EEG, but MEG has the ability to capture activity originating deep within the brain that often cannot be seen with the EEG. The MEG is a very expensive machine valued at millions of dollars, which is why it's only available at a few epilepsy centers in the world. However, it may certainly be worth the cost, as it can be of great help in identifying a seizure focus.

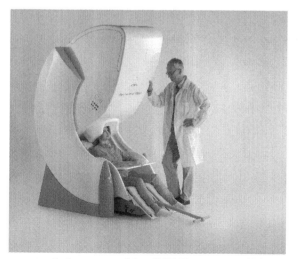

Magnetoencephalogram machine (MEG) courtesy of Elekta, corp

- **Test - Imaging Studies**

It's often necessary to create a "picture" of the brain itself, and for that we turn to imaging studies. The images produced by these studies can reveal malformations, brain damage and other abnormalities that may be causing the seizures.

There are several ways to produce images of the brain, including computed tomography (CT), magnetic resonance imaging (MRI), PET scans, SPECT scans, and MR spectroscopy (MRS).

Computed tomography (CT)

CT is an x-ray that provides two-dimensional and three-dimensional cross-sectional images of the brain. On a CT scan, most kinds of brain abnormalities, like tumors, evidence of stroke, malformations or infections will be clearly visible. Used in conjunction with an EEG, the CT scan provides a picture of the brain, while the EEG shows the distribution of electrical activity. Because the CT scan emits a small amount of radiation, it should be avoided during pregnancy.

Magnetic resonance imaging (MRI)

An MRI creates a magnetic field that provides a more detailed picture of the brain. Sequences of pictures of the brain called "brain cuts" are taken to view possible areas of seizure origin in greater detail. The high-resolution MRI offers a more sophisticated view of the brain with additional details, compared to the standard MRI and CT. Because of its magnetic field, MRIs should be avoided by those who have metal parts in their bodies (surgical clips, staples, artificial joints, shunts, vein filters, stimulators, shrapnel, etc.) as it could cause severe internal damage in those areas. To date there has been no indication that the use of MRI during pregnancy has produced negative effects.

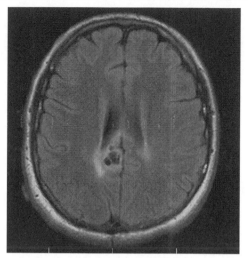

MRI revealing brain tumor on the right side of the brain

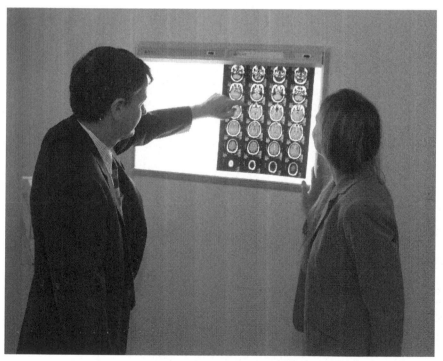

Neurologists specializing in epilepsy reviewing MRI findings

Positron emission tomography (PET scan)

The PET scan measures the amount of fuel (glucose) that the brain uses. In those with partial epilepsy, seizures may be originating in a damaged area that has fewer viable brain cells. Because it has fewer cells, that area might consume less glucose or none at all. This can be detected on the PET scan and point toward the seizure focus. For the scan, a tracer containing a dye combined with glucose is injected when the patient is *not* having a seizure, to monitor the way in which glucose is taken up by different parts of the brain. Any part of the brain that takes up less glucose than expected may be the seizure focus.

Single photon emission computed tomography (SPECT scan)

A SPECT scan measures the amount of blood that goes to different parts of the brain. During a partial seizure, extra blood will travel to the "seizure area," as the brain cells there need more oxygen and glucose. If the patient is having a seizure, doctors can perform a SPECT scan to identify areas of the brain that have increased blood flow. For the SPECT scan a tracer is injected *while* the patient is having a seizure. A separate study is also performed while the patient is *not* having a seizure, and the results of the two scans are compared to show the difference in blood flow.

MR spectroscopy (MRS)

MRS measures small chemical compounds produced by the brain called metabolites. The three main metabolites measured are n-acetyl aspartate (NAA), which gives a reading of the amounts of brain cells, and choline and creatine, which indicate the amount of scar tissue and thus, brain damage. If there is no damage to the brain, the level of NAA will be greater than the choline/creatine levels. If brain damage *is* present, there will be less NAA and more choline/creatine.

49

Genetic Testing For Epilepsy

For some patients, genetic testing can help guide therapy and determine the long-term prognosis. Genetic tests for epilepsy are still being developed and guidelines as to who should be tested, when the test should take place, or which test to order are not developed yet. An exception is those with epilepsy-related developmental delays, who might benefit from a microscopic examination of their chromosomes or various tests that show how certain genes are functioning. Be aware, however, that many genetic tests are very expensive and may not be covered by insurance.

The most common motivation for genetic testing for epilepsy is to see if the disorder might be passed on to future children. Yet a diagnosis of epilepsy is never a reason to keep from having children. Although children of a parent who has epilepsy do have a slightly higher risk of developing the disorder, the vast majority will not. And those who do inherit epilepsy are usually blessed with normal intellectual ability, a good response to seizure medications and (sometimes) remission after childhood. However, family counseling should be considered for those with certain rare familial causes of epilepsy such as tuberous sclerosis, as there is a high risk of passing it to their children.

Because there is no one-size-fits-all answer to "Should I have a genetic test?", my best advice is discuss the pros and cons with your doctor and make the decision accordingly.

CLASSIFYING EPILEPSY

Once your doctor has determined that you do have epilepsy, he or she will classify it according to cause and type.

- *Cause* – As noted in Chapter 2, the cause of epilepsy is either *idiopathic* (unknown) or *symptomatic* (known). An example of an idiopathic cause is genetics, while symptomatic causes include head injuries, strokes, brain tumors, infections, malformations and problems during pregnancy and delivery.

- *Type* – The type of seizure falls into one of two major categories: *generalized* (meaning the seizure involves the entire brain) or *partial* (the seizure involves just a part of the brain).

There are only four combinations of cause and type. They are *idiopathic generalized, idiopathic partial, symptomatic generalized* and *symptomatic partial*. The classification can be further refined according to the specific symptoms of the seizures (aura, muscle contractions, childhood-onset, and so on), producing a large number of different types of epilepsy. Below is a brief description of the four cause/type combinations. They will be described in greater detail in Chapter 4: The Epilepsy Syndromes.

Idiopathic Generalized Epilepsy

The cause of these seizures is unknown and they affect the entire brain. Some of these disorders are believed to be strongly related to genetics, and they typically occur any time between infancy and the end of adolescence. There may be jerking of the extremities (myoclonic seizures), staring spells (absence seizures) or "grand mal" seizures (tonic-clonic seizures). Some types are eventually outgrown. The idiopathic generalized epilepsies include:

- **Benign neonatal familial convulsions**

- **Benign myoclonic epilepsy of infancy**

- **Generalized epilepsy with febrile seizures plus**

- **Epilepsy with myoclonic absences**

- **Epilepsy with myoclonic-astatic seizures**

- Childhood absence epilepsy ("petit mal epilepsy")

- Juvenile absence epilepsy ("petit mal epilepsy")

- Juvenile myoclonic epilepsy

- Epilepsy with generalized tonic-clonic seizures only ("grand mal epilepsy")

Idiopathic Partial Epilepsy

The cause is unknown and the seizures affect just a part of the brain. Types of idiopathic partial epilepsies include:

- Benign rolandic epilepsy

- Benign occipital epilepsy

Symptomatic Generalized Epilepsy

The cause is known or highly suspected and seizures affect the entire brain. Cerebral palsy and/or mental delay may also be present. There can be many types of seizures, including atypical absence, tonic, myoclonic and generalized tonic-clonic. Types of symptomatic generalized epilepsies include:

- Infantile spasms (West syndrome)

- Dravet syndrome

- Lennox-Gastaut epilepsy

Symptomatic Partial Epilepsies

The cause is known – an abnormality in a specific area (lobe) of the brain, or a combination of lobes – and seizures affect a part of the brain. Since each lobe has a different function, the symptoms will depend on the lobe that is affected. This type of epilepsy is most likely to begin in adults, although children can also be affected. Types of symptomatic partial epilepsies include:

- **Temporal lobe epilepsy** - affecting memory, smell, hearing, automatic behaviors and understanding of language (if it is dominant brain hemisphere-usually the left in right handed individuals)

- **Frontal lobe epilepsy** - affecting movement, planning, social skills and expression of language (if it is the dominant brain hemisphere-usually the left is right handed individuals)

- **Parietal lobe epilepsy** - affecting touch and other sensations on the skin

- **Occipital lobe epilepsy** - affecting the visual center of the brain

(For a more complete description of symptomatic partial epilepsy seizures and their symptoms, see Appendix 3 - Symptomatic Partial Epilepsies by Lobe.)

Special Types of Epilepsy

Not all seizures fall easily into the categories of partial or generalized. Some are different from the rest; they may be partial *and* generalized, affect the speech, start in one part of the brain and spread, or vice versa. These special types of epilepsy include:

- **Neonatal seizures** – This disorder is characterized by seizures in newborn babies. Because the symptoms are subtle and may not differ much from typical infant behavior, they may not be recognized as seizure behaviors. Symptoms include continuous sucking, chewing or drooling, repetitive eye movements, blinking or fluttering of the eyelids, a fixed gaze toward one side, stepping movements of the legs, rowing movements of the arms and/or jerking muscles. Seizures occur more frequently in newborn babies (especially those who are premature) than in any other segment of the population. Over half of the infants who have neonatal seizures will develop epilepsy later in life.

- **Landau-Kleffner syndrome** – This rare disorder affects areas of the child's brain that govern speech and comprehension. The child will usually develop normal language skills then lose them between the ages of 3 and 8. Seizures may or may not occur. Landau-Kleffner syndrome is often mistaken for autism, ADD, learning disorders or emotional problems.

- **ESES (electrical status epilepticus during sleep)** – Another rare disorder affecting children, ESES typically occurs in children who have already been diagnosed with epilepsy. There may be difficulty in understanding or expressing language or with the thought process. There may be absence seizures while the child is awake, or myoclonic seizures, particularly during the night when the child is asleep. An EEG shows continuous spike and wave activity during sleep, particularly during a period called "slow wave" sleep.

- **Reflex epilepsy** – In this condition, seizures can occur in response to external stimuli or, less often, internal mental processes. In the most common type, photosensitive epilepsy, a seizure can occur in response to visual stimuli such as flashing lights or rapidly alternating light and dark patterns. Being immersed in hot water, reading, listening to music or hearing a certain tone of voice can stimulate seizures in some people with reflex epilepsy.

BEGINNING THE TREATMENT

Once your doctor has completed testing and diagnosed your specific type of epilepsy, your path to good health will become much clearer. Treatments may include medication(s), surgery, special diets, various alternative or complementary therapies or some combination of these. Most likely, your doctor will begin by giving you some form of medication. In Chapter 6, you'll learn about the anti-epileptic drugs (AEDs) and how they work. But as I've said before, medications are only part of the comprehensive, well-rounded treatment program discussed in this book that addresses the physical, emotional, lifestyle and other issues related to epilepsy. It's all important!

CHAPTER FOUR
THE EPILEPSY SYNDROMES

As you learned in the last chapter, the proper classification of epilepsy types is very important in the treatment and management of the disorder. And it can also provide vital information for *you*. When you thoroughly understand the kind of epilepsy that's affecting you (or your child), you'll have a much better idea of what you can expect in terms of symptoms, intensity and duration. For example, did you know that some types of epilepsy can be outgrown, while others last for a lifetime? That medication may not be needed in some cases, as the seizures occur infrequently and don't cause significant risk? Or in other cases, that skipping medication can be life threatening or make a child much more likely to develop learning problems and developmental delay? It pays to learn all you can about epilepsy and how to keep it under good control.

This chapter will give you a crash course in the various types of epilepsy, their symptoms, treatment and prognosis. I've arranged it according to the age at which the seizures first occurred, as age plays a crucial role in the development and outcome of the disorder.

NEWBORN PERIOD

Because the brain in a baby or young child is growing rapidly and making new connections between neurons, it is more vulnerable to electrical overload, which makes it more seizure-prone. This is especially true if there is an additional irritant or provocation like a fever, infection or injury. In addition, a baby's brain waves change rapidly during the first few weeks of life, increasing the risk of certain types of seizures that cannot occur in the brain of an older child or adult. For these reasons, seizures occur more frequently in newborn babies (especially those who are premature) than in any other segment of the population. And, it's a sad fact that over half of newborns who have seizures will develop epilepsy later in life.

The seizures in newborns can take many forms, including clonic (repeated rhythmic jerking of one or more limb), tonic (sudden stiff posture), or subtle seizures (staring, or repeated non-purposeful movements like sucking or "bicycling" foot movements) and fall into the category of idiopathic (no obvious cause) or symptomatic (the cause is known).

Idiopathic Neonatal Convulsions

These seizures occur in otherwise healthy newborns during the first two weeks of life. The EEG patterns (brain waves) are normal or relatively normal between seizures and the overall prognosis is good. Tests must be performed to rule out infection of the brain, brain injury including stroke, or a metabolic cause, as these conditions can be life threatening and will require immediate intervention.

If no cause can be found despite a complete evaluation, the seizures are classified as idiopathic and further defined as either *benign familial neonatal convulsions* or *benign idiopathic neonatal convulsions*.

- **Benign familial neonatal convulsions** – These seizures typically occur in first 2-15 days of life and are usually clonic (rhythmic jerking of one or both arms and legs), but they may start with more subtle actions such as staring, chewing movements or an unusual cry. The seizures start from either side of the brain, often alternating from the left to the right with subsequent episodes. Seizures typically occur immediately after waking from sleep.

Typically there is a history of seizures occurring during the first two weeks of life in either the mother or the father; possibly in the grandparents. Although these infants may have many seizures per day (as many as several per hour), the prognosis is good. They usually develop normally, eat appropriately, spend a normal amount of time asleep and awake, and exhibit alertness when awake. No medications are needed.

- **Benign idiopathic neonatal convulsions (also called Fifth Day Fits)** – Seizures often begin on or around the fifth day after birth. They are usually either clonic (rhythmic jerking of one or more arms and/or legs) or apneic (baby briefly stops breathing). There may be a dramatic color change in which the infant becomes very pale or even looks bluish in color. Most will outgrow the seizures and have normal development and intelligence in the future; rarely there may be some developmental delay. No medications are needed.

Symptomatic Neonatal Convulsions

These seizures, which are usually due to birth asphyxia, bleeding, stroke or infection, may be temporary or the first sign of a serious epilepsy syndrome, in which other types of epilepsy develop during infancy or early childhood. The seizures often occur within a few hours of delivery or after a bleed or a stroke, and EEG monitoring shows very abnormal brain waves. Symptomatic neonatal convulsions include:

- **Tonic seizures** - Characterized by sudden sustained stiffening and posturing of the arms and body.

- **Myoclonic seizures** – Characterized by sudden quick random jerks of different limbs.

These convulsions may be difficult to control during the first hours or days of life. For some babies, the seizures can be well controlled after a few days. Then, after a few days to a few months of treatment, the doctor may decide that seizure medications can be stopped. For those who have a metabolic disorder, certain dietary restrictions may be indicated. But for those who have hard-to-control seizures that last into infancy and early childhood, often due to brain malformations or genetic/metabolic disorders, the seizures may be very difficult to control with medications. In such cases, surgery may be recommended.

EARLY INFANCY

Infantile Spasms (West Syndrome)
These very brief, convulsive movements, which typically occur in clusters, consist of dramatic, rapid, forward or backward bending of the neck, trunk, arms and/or legs. A more subtle form consists of a sudden, brief head drop. An EEG will reveal disorganized brain activity with scattered spikes between events, then a sudden flattening during the spasm.

Infantile spasms occur during the first year of life, typically between 3 and 9 months, and can have a profoundly negative influence on a child's development. Nearly 45% will have significant intellectual disabilities, although a small percentage with no identifiable cause of the disease will be intellectually normal. Approximately one-third of cases will progress to Lennox Gastaut Syndrome (described in section on Late Infancy).

There are numerous causes, identifiable in about 70 percent of cases. They include structural abnormalities of the brain (smooth brain, cortex malformation, abnormal fluid space); Down's syndrome; tuberous sclerosis; neurofibromatosis; vitamin B6 deficiency; birth injury (lack of oxygen or blood to the brain); and meningitis or encephalitis contracted in utero or after birth. A physical examination including the skin is very important as some causes (tuberous sclerosis and neurofibromatosis) can be identified by hallmark signs such as reddish spots on the nose and cheeks in a butterfly pattern, light patches on the skin, small tumors around the toenails or fingernails, and so on.

The prognosis is highly dependent on the underlying cause. For example, a child who has infantile spasms due to severe, irreversible brain injury will not be expected to improve. But one who has the condition due to vitamin B6 deficiency may experience a complete reversal of the disease with vitamin therapy. As for other causes, isolated structural abnormalities such as cortical dysplasia can be treated surgically. Infantile spasms in patients with tuberous sclerosis have been shown to respond particularly well to vigabatrin (Sabril®). Adrenocorticotropic hormone (ACTH) can help control the seizures, but it is unknown if it will improve the child's long-term cognitive outcome. And a ketogenic diet has recently been shown to be effective in many cases of infantile spasms. (See Chapter 8: Diet Therapy.) More studies need to be done to find the most effective treatment for individual cases of infantile spasms.

Benign Myoclonic Epilepsy of Infancy
Characterized by sudden, quick, random jerks of the limbs, these seizures occur in children ages 6 months to 3 years. Thirty percent of them are triggered by lights or being startled; others may occur with fever (febrile seizures). On an EEG, benign myoclonic epilepsy of infancy is associated with a polyspike wave during the seizure with normal brain waves in between seizures. The cause is unknown.

In most cases, the prognosis is good: physical and mental development are normal. Rarely there can be a predisposition toward tonic-clonic ("grand mal") seizures later in life. Treatment usually consists of valproic acid (Depakote®), but only for a few years.

Severe Myoclonic Epilepsy of Infancy (Dravet Syndrome)

This severe form of epilepsy begins at around one year of age in the form of prolonged febrile (fever-related) seizures. Later, generalized tonic-clonic ("grand mal") seizures, atypical absence seizures and complex partial seizures may also occur. Status epilepticus (uncontrolled, continuous seizure) may also occur. In up to 80 percent of cases, the cause of Dravet syndrome is a defect in a gene necessary for brain cell function. Associated problems include autism, movement disorders, upper respiratory infections, sleep disorders, problems with nutrition and growth, and sudden unexplained death in epilepsy (SUDEP). There is also an increased risk of intellectual disability that correlates with seizure frequency, and epilepsy that persists into adulthood.

While Dravet syndrome is difficult to control, seizures can be reduced with anti-epileptic medications and, possibly, a ketogenic diet. Typically, the seizures become less severe or disappear over time, and 85 percent of patients survive to adulthood.

Generalized Epilepsies with Febrile Seizures Plus (GEFS+)

Those with GEFS+ come from families with epilepsy that affects members from different generations. In any family member, the first sign is usually febrile (fever related) seizures. While febrile seizures usually occur only in those under the age of 6, in GEFS+ families they can occur beyond that age (a major clue for diagnosing this syndrome). Other seizure types seen in these families include absence, myoclonic, generalized tonic-clonic and atonic.

The cause of GEFS+ is genetic, and several slight genetic abnormalities can be detected through blood tests. Because so many different forms of seizures are associated with this syndrome, prognosis and treatment depend on the type of seizures experienced.

LATE INFANCY

Lennox-Gastaut Syndrome (LSG)

The first signs of this severe form of epilepsy usually occur between ages 2 and 8 and one-third of the time they are preceded by infantile spasms. The types of seizures vary in LGS, but may include tonic, atonic, atypical absence, generalized tonic-clonic and multifocal partial. Status epilepticus (prolonged seizure) is common and can take many different forms. For example, there may be prolonged atypical absence seizures easily mistaken for slow thinking/responsiveness.

LGS is usually associated with some level of impaired intellectual function, developmental delay and behavioral issues. An EEG shows a classic pattern of slow spike and wave. The syndrome can stem from various causes including structural abnormalities of the brain (smooth brain, cortex malformation or abnormal fluid space), infection affecting the brain (meningitis or encephalitis) in utero or after birth, lack of blood or oxygen to the brain causing brain damage and various metabolic causes. Genetic causes are rare.

As for the prognosis, cognitive deterioration may occur and seizures tend to be treatment-resistant. The likelihood of epilepsy remission is very low. Treatment includes many anti-epileptic medications, with more success seen with felbamate (Felbatol®), plus co-management by a team of specialists including behaviorists and child mental health providers.

CHILDHOOD

Childhood Absence Epilepsy

The most common form of childhood epilepsy, absence seizures (also known as "petit mal" seizures) are brief periods during which the child becomes unaware of the environment and stares blankly into the distance. The seizures usually begin in children age 4 to 10 years and can occur very frequently and in clusters. Known triggers of absence seizures include hyperventilation and, more rarely, photic stimulation (flashing or flickering lights). The characteristic EEG for childhood absence epilepsy shows a pattern known as generalized 3 Hz spike-wave discharges.

The cause of this form of epilepsy is most likely genetic, as most have a family history of epilepsy. Treatment generally involves one of the anti-epileptic medications, such as valproic acid (Depakote®), ethosuximide (Zarontin®), lamotrigine (Lamictal®), or levetiracetam (Keppra®) among others. In 70 percent of cases, childhood absence epilepsy disappears during adolescence. The child's physical/mental development is normal. In some, however, generalized tonic-clonic ("grand mal") seizures occur later in life

Epilepsy with Myoclonic Absences

This syndrome, which typically starts around the age of 7, includes rhythmic jerking of the shoulders, arms and legs accompanied by muscle contraction, usually in the shoulders or deltoid muscles, which may elevate the arms. These seizures occur several times a day and can last from 10 to 60 seconds. The typical EEG shows a generalized, rhythmic 3 Hz spike-wave or a polyspike-wave.

The cause is unknown, although in about 25 percent of cases there is a family history of seizures. About half the time this form of epilepsy disappears after about 5 years; otherwise, it continues into adulthood. Treatment usually consists of valproic acid (Depakote®) and ethosuximide (Zarontin®), although other newer medications may also be of help.

Epilepsy with Myoclonic-Astatic Seizures

There is a unique feature to these seizures, which typically begin by the age of 5: after a short period of jerking of the shoulders, arms and or legs, the supporting muscles suddenly go limp. The legs can give way or the body may suddenly slump. If standing, the child may fall heavily (known as a "drop attack") and hit the ground with a violent impact. Since these seizures typically happen several times a day, they present an ongoing risk of persistent, major injury. Other seizures may also be present, including absence, tonic-clonic ("grand mal") and non-convulsive status epilepticus.

There is no known cause for myoclonic-astatic seizures, although it affects three times as many boys as girls and there appears to be a strong genetic link. Many children outgrow these seizures, although some remain treatment resistant and might experience some degree of developmental delay. Valproic acid (Depakote®) is typically used for treatment, however newer medications like lamotrigine (Lamictal®), levetiracetam (Keppra®) or others may be used when there is resistance to the first medication.

Landau Kleffner Syndrome (Acquired Epileptic Aphasia)

In this rare neurological disorder, a child develops normal speech and language skills then, sometime between ages 3 and 8, suddenly or gradually loses the ability to understand or express language (a condition called aphasia). Atypical absence or generalized tonic-clonic seizures precede the loss of language in 7 out of 10 patients.

While often misdiagnosed as hearing loss, autism, a learning disability or mental retardation, Landau Kleffner syndrome is actually a problem in processing information. The cause is unclear. On an EEG, there will be spikes in the temporal region of the brain that are more active when the child has aphasia.

Treatment for Landau Kleffner syndrome may include anti-epileptic medications such as valproic acid (Depakote®), ethosuximide (Zarontin®), benzodiazepines, steroids or gamma globulin (a protein in the blood plasma that includes antibodies). In some cases, surgery may be performed that cuts nerve fibers in the outer layers of the brain without affecting the deeper layers that govern vital functions (this surgery is called "Multiple Subpial Transections"). In most cases, treatment strategies result in good seizure control. Speech may or may not improve.

Benign Rolandic Epilepsy (BRE)

This syndrome characterized by brief, partial seizures affecting the face and mouth account for 15-20 percent of childhood epilepsies. BRE strikes children 3 to 13 years old, most frequently between ages 7 and 8. Typically, episodes occur at night during sleep or immediately upon awakening and manifest as jerking or tingling sensations in the mouth, difficulty talking and increased drooling. An EEG shows sharp waves over the central and temporal regions of the brain that are much more apparent during sleep.

Named after an area in the brain called the rolandic strip (or "motor strip"), BRE is considered "benign" because it rarely causes harm, does not affect intelligence, is not due to structural problems in the brain, and is usually outgrown by adolescence. The genetic component is strong: approximately 40 percent of those affected have close relatives with this form of epilepsy.

Treatment is typically not required unless the seizures become repetitive, affect cognition or occur during wakefulness. Prognosis for this kind of epilepsy is very good to excellent. Brain development generally remains normal (although in some cases there are mild cognitive problems), and the seizures typically disappear by the time the child becomes an adolescent.

Benign Occipital Epilepsy - Childhood Epilepsy with Occipital Paroxysms (CEOP)

These seizure syndromes are so-named because their EEGs show long runs of high magnitude, repetitive spikes that originate from the occipital lobe of the brain, the visual processing center. There are two distinct types of CEOP, which are defined according to the age they first occur: early-onset and late-onset.

- **Early-Onset Childhood Occipital Epilepsy (*Panayiotopoulos syndrome*)** – In this form of epilepsy the seizures first occur around the age of 5 and often stop at about age 6. Most seizures occur during sleep and the symptoms are vomiting and temporary loss of consciousness. There may also be eye deviation (eyes moving to one side in a forced manner), and the seizure could evolve into a generalized tonic-clonic seizure with a loss of consciousness. In 3 out of 10 children, the seizure goes on long enough to be considered status epilepticus. In most, an EEG shows high voltage spikes in the occipital area of the brain.

Generally, no treatment is necessary and the prognosis is excellent. One-third of patients have just one seizure, while half have two to five. Seizures usually disappear within two years and the chance of developing adult seizures is no greater than the risk seen in the general population. If treatment is needed, carbamazepine (Tegretol®) or lamotrigine (Lamictal®) are the medications most commonly used, although other medications may also be of help.

- **Late-Onset Childhood Occipital Epilepsy (*Gastaut Syndrome*)** – These seizures, which usually begin between the age of 8 and 10, are much more frequent than the early-onset type, occurring every day and sometimes more than once a day. They typically begin with visual hallucinations or spells of blindness that last 3-5 minutes, and there may be eye pain, repetitive blinking and eyelid fluttering. A clonic seizure involving half of the body ensues, lasting less than a minute – and sometimes only seconds usually follows. After the seizure, there may be headaches similar to migraines, which can interfere with proper diagnosis. As with early-onset, the EEG of late-onset childhood occipital epilepsy shows high amplitude spikes in the occipital area of the brain.

The late-onset form, like early-onset childhood occipital epilepsy, stems from genetic causes; however the prognosis is not as favorable. Although many children will outgrow the seizures, some may experience them in adulthood and seizure control may be difficult. Carbamazepine (Tegretol®) is usually the medication of choice.

ESES (Electrical Status Epilepticus During Sleep)

This rare disorder stemming from unknown causes usually occurs in mid-childhood in those who have already been diagnosed with epilepsy. The first signs may be difficulties with understanding language or expressing thoughts, and a significant slowdown in the rate of learning. There may be absence, myoclonic among other seizures. An EEG shows continuous spike and wave activity during sleep, especially during the period called "slow wave" sleep.

These seizures usually disappear by the mid-teens but most children do not return to normal levels in language and attention skills. While seizures are present, the medications typically used to control them include clobazam (Frisium®), ethosuximide (Zarontin®) and valproic acid (Depakote®); newer medications may also help.

Reflex Epilepsy

These seizures typically occur in response to external stimuli. In the most common type of reflex epilepsy, photosensitive epilepsy, seizures are brought on by flashing lights, rapidly alternating light and dark patterns or other visual stimuli. But in some cases, seizures can occur in response to internal mental processes, like reading, listening to music or hearing a certain tone of voice. About 85 percent of the seizures are generalized tonic-clonic ("grand mal"), but absence seizures and myoclonic (jerking) seizures can also occur.

Photosensitive epilepsy usually starts during childhood and some, but not all, children will outgrow it by adulthood. In the meantime, because it's difficult to avoid the kinds of stimulation that bring on these seizures, medications are usually required, typically valproic acid (Depakote®), clonazepam (Klonopin®) or clobazam (Frisium®); newer medications may also help.

LATE CHILDHOOD - ADOLESCENCE

Juvenile Absence Epilepsy

These absence seizures are similar to those experienced in childhood absence epilepsy, but are milder and less frequent. They first appear around the age of puberty. Generalized tonic-clonic ("grand mal") seizures occur in 80 percent of those with juvenile absence epilepsy, and about 20 percent experience occasional myoclonic jerking. Juvenile absence epilepsy shows the same EEG pattern seen in childhood absence epilepsy, 3Hz generalized spike-wave discharges. Genetics are the most likely cause; a family history of epilepsy is seen in about 11 percent of patients.

The most common trigger for juvenile absence epilepsy is hyperventilation, followed by mental or psychological stress. Sleep deprivation, alcohol and photic stimulation (flashing or flickering lights) can also be precipitating factors.

While juvenile absence epilepsy could be a lifelong disorder, seizures can be controlled in about 85 percent of patients using one of the following anti-epileptic medications: valproic acid (Depakote®), lamotrigine (Lamictal®), ethosuximide (Zarontin®) or levetiracetam (Keppra®). Fifteen percent will require more than one anti-epileptic medication. Other medications could also be of help.

Juvenile Myoclonic Epilepsy

This common form of epilepsy, characterized by myoclonic seizures (jerking of the arms, shoulders or legs) usually occurs for the first time between ages 12 and 18. The seizures typically strike in the morning, just after awakening. About 80 percent of the time generalized tonic-clonic seizure ("grand mal") also occur, and around 20% will also have absence seizures. On an EEG, there are generalized polyspike-wave discharges.

Juvenile myoclonic seizures can be triggered by photic stimulation (flashing or flickering lights), sleep deprivation or hyperventilation. The most likely cause is genetics, as about 50 percent of patients have a family history of epilepsy.

Although juvenile myoclonic epilepsy is easy to control, it requires treatment for life. The medications typically used include valproic acid (Depakote®), lamotrigine (Lamictal®), levetiracetam (Keppra®), topiramate (Topamax®) and zonisamide (Zonegran®).

Generalized Tonic-Clonic Seizures on Awakening (GTC on Awakening)

GTC on awakening typically begins sometime around adolescence and consists of "grand mal" seizures that occur upon awakening (after napping or a night's sleep), although the seizures can also occur in the evening when drowsiness sets in. GTC on awakening is often seen in conjunction with myoclonic seizures or absence seizures, which can occur one after another (e.g. the jerking movements of myoclonic seizures may be immediately followed by a tonic-clonic seizure, which is followed by an absence seizure), or as single events. An EEG will show generalized spike-wave discharges.

Genetics are most likely responsible for GTC on awakening, with a family history of epilepsy seen in 12 percent of patients. Triggers include photic stimulation (flickering or flashing lights), sleep deprivation and excessive alcohol intake.

The prognosis for this syndrome is very good as it is easy to control with valproic acid (Depakote®). However it does require treatment for life. Newer medications can also be helpful.

THE IMPORTANCE OF KNOWING

As you can see, correctly pinpointing the epilepsy syndrome that is affecting you (or your child) is crucial, as all of these syndromes have different characteristics, treatments and outcomes. Diagnosis is the fulcrum; all treatments and therapies stem from that one decision, so it must be correct. Now that you know the general characteristics of each of these epilepsy syndromes, you can provide the treatment team with valuable information by carefully noting any signs and symptoms, reactions to medications, psychological states and so on related to the seizures. Your input will help the doctor zero in on the diagnosis and may make the difference between a successful and an unsuccessful treatment. So stay aware, be vigilant and take notes! As the Chinese general Sun Tzu said in his famous book, *The Art of War*, "If you know your enemies and know yourself, you will not be imperiled in a hundred battles; if you do not know your enemies nor yourself, you will be imperiled in every single battle."

CHAPTER FIVE
TREATMENT & PREVENTION

The goal of epilepsy treatment is to diminish/prevent future seizures via medication, surgery and/or other means, and address the psychological problems and other complications that stem from the disorder. Briefly put, the treatment steps are:

1. **Work with your doctor, educating him/her about yourself and your symptoms and learning all you can from her/him about the disorder and how to help yourself**

2. **Avoid triggers for your seizures**

3. **Use the appropriate medication(s)**

4. **Consider following an "anti-epilepsy" diet**

5. **Eliminate the seizure focus through surgery, if necessary**

6. **Explore supportive, complementary and experimental treatments**

For a small number of people with mild seizures well-controlled by medicine with no accompanying physical or psychological distress, medications may be enough. But most patients need a comprehensive approach to treatment that encompasses both mind and body (i.e. medicine and psychology), and offers support for dealing with the practical, social and legal issues that arise. Let's take a closer look at each of these steps.

STEP #1: WORK WITH YOUR DOCTOR

In days not too long past, the doctor was treated as an all-knowing demi-god, and the patient was expected to be passive and accept any treatments offered. Asking questions was considered odd, if not downright annoying, and the answers given were often short and uninformative.

Fortunately, now that's all changed because we've learned that people tend to do better when they actively participate in their treatment. This is especially true for epilepsy, which has no simple, one-size-fits-all cure. Thus it's vitally important that you work closely with your doctor so a tailor-made treatment can be created to suit your special needs.

This process of collaboration begins during your search for the "right" doctor. "Right" can be hard to define when personality factors enter the equation, as they likely will. But it is possible to define "right" in terms of what the doctor can offer you. A large number of epilepsy patients are *not* treated by specialists who have spent years studying the disorder and working with epilepsy patients. While doctors that do not specialize in epilepsy may be able to help you, they are most likely not geared toward handling all aspects of epilepsy. That's why you might want to look for an epileptologist, the kind of doctor specifically trained to help you control your epilepsy. Of course, it's possible that you live in an area where there are no epileptologists. If this is the case, I suggest you find a doctor who specializes in neurology.

Searching For the "Right" Doctor

Before agreeing to become anyone's patient, consider these questions:

- Does the doctor have the right training and expertise? An epileptologist is preferable. (See box below: "Aren't All Doctors Qualified to Treat Epilepsy?")
- Is the doctor part of a medical group? This is important, as a solo practitioner may not be available when you need help most (unless she/he has proper coverage).

- Is the medical group available 24/7?

- Does the medical group provide programs specific to your needs? These may include:

  o diet program

  o stimulator program

  o surgical program

  o experimental drugs program

- Does the medical group provide other services that can help improve your quality of life? These may include:

  o support groups

  o therapy for anxiety, depression and related ailments

  o memory remediation programs to improve day-to-day functioning

  o wellness resources

- If you call after hours, will an attending epileptologist be available to take care of your problems or answer your questions? Or will you be talking to a doctor-in-training?

Most groups do not provide direct access to your personal doctor unless he/she happens to be on call that day. This means you'll talk to the doctor who is "on call." Some epilepsy groups have epilepsy specialists covering after hours, but in many institutions there are only trainees (such as residents or fellows). This is an important question to ask and could be a deciding factor when choosing a doctor.

Aren't All Doctors Qualified to Treat Epilepsy?

The short answer to this question is "yes" in the sense that every physician, whether an M.D. (medical doctor) or D.O. (doctor of osteopathy), has graduated from medical school and is legally qualified to treat people with epilepsy. However, most M.D.s and D.O.s have *not* had additional training in the recognition and management of this disorder.

Doctors who treat epilepsy vary in their levels of sophistication regarding the disorder. The first level consists of primary care physicians, such as pediatricians, internists or family doctors, who have had no additional training specific to neurology or epilepsy.

The second level consists of general neurologists specializing in diseases of the nervous system, which includes the brain. They have had four years of post-medical school training in neurology, and many are also Board Certified in Neurology.

The third level consists of epileptologists, who are neurologists who specialize in the treatment of epilepsy. Epileptologists are experts in seizure disorders, special conditions involving seizures, and the use of anticonvulsants and other treatments. Epileptologists have received the same training as general neurologists, plus up to three additional years of training in epilepsy, and many are Board Certified in Clinical Neurophysiology/ Epilepsy.

Although there are very competent and experienced physicians to be found in all three levels, if your epilepsy is not under control, you'll be better off with an epileptologist who has spent years mastering the diagnosis and treatment of epilepsy.

Does the Doctor "Feel" Right?

Just because a doctor is highly qualified and belongs to a top medical group offering every service you'll ever need doesn't mean that he/ she is right for you. If you don't feel comfortable with the doctor and the medical staff, look for another doctor. There's nothing specific that you can measure; it's simply a matter of intuition and feelings. Some helpful questions to ask yourself after meeting a prospective doctor include:

- Did the doctor answer all of my questions?

- Did I feel rushed during the appointment?

- Was the staff polite, friendly and competent?

- Did I feel calm and well cared for?

- Did the doctor make me wait long past my appointment time before seeing me?

- Did the doctor seem to value my input, curiosity and seriousness about my condition?

- Did the doctor treat me like a partner?

- Did I feel comfortable asking questions and divulging personal information?

- Did I feel like I couldn't wait to get out of the doctor's office?

Your honest answers to these questions should help you decide whether or not you want this doctor to spearhead your treatment. If you decide this is not the person for you, keep looking. The right doctor is out there.

The Initial Examination

Once you've decided on a doctor, you'll make an initial appointment. During this appointment, the doctor will compile a great deal of information about you, your medical history, family medical history and symptoms. You will provide more accurate information if you write down your medical history, family medical history, symptoms and everything you can remember about your seizures (including what went on immediately beforehand).

It's also a good idea to bring along a family member or friend who has witnessed the seizures, as most patients do not recall their seizures or all of the events leading up to them. And be sure to bring your medical records and any test results, along with any medications that you're taking *in their containers*. (A lot of important information is listed on the container label.)

Once the doctor has performed an initial evaluation, it's your turn to ask questions such as:

- Do I have epilepsy?

- What type of epilepsy do I have?

- Will I need further testing in order to clarify my type of epilepsy?

- Why do I have epilepsy?

- Do I need to do something in particular to avoid seizures?

- What should be done when I have a seizure?

- What are the treatment options and potential complications of each one?

- Which support services do you recommend?

Possibilities may include:

  o support groups

  o memory treatment programs

  o psychotherapy

- Are these support services available in your group?

- What do I tell my family and friends?

- What do I tell my employer?

- How is this going to affect my

  o driving

  o working

  o relationships

  o children

  o quality of life

Don't be afraid to speak up! Many patients are nervous about questioning their doctors, fearing they will either be ignored or won't understand the answers. If you're ignored, ask again. And if you don't understand the answer, ask for clarification. You certainly want to respect the doctor's time, but remember that the time you spend with the doctor is *your* time.

Follow-Up Visits

Once treatment begins, you'll see your doctor regularly for follow-up visits. During these visits, the doctor will ask about any seizures you may have had, their strength and type; as well as medication side effects and any other problems you may be having.

As soon as possible you should start to keep a seizure calendar. On this calendar, note when each seizure occurred, where you were, how long it lasted and anything you think may be relevant. These factors could include stressors, family events, lack of sleep, menses, exposure to flashing lights and so on. Bring the calendar with you when you visit the doctor to help determine seizure frequency, seizure strength and the factors that may be triggering them. You should also note any medication side effects, including what they were, when they occurred and how long they lasted.

Once the doctor has recorded this information and performed any necessary tests, it will be your turn to ask questions such as:

- Is treatment going as well as you hoped for?

- Will I need further testing?

- Is my current medication still the most appropriate one for me?

- Are there other alternative treatments?

- Do you think I could benefit from supportive measures (a support group, memory treatment, psychotherapy, epilepsy walks, volunteering)?

To ensure a smooth question-and-answer session, write out your questions ahead of time. Doing so will help you sort through important issues and ensure that you don't forget them when you're in the doctor's presence. It's also helpful to take notes during your visit so you can remember the answers.

What to Do Between Visits

During the time that you're on your own, be sure to follow your doctor's instructions carefully, take your medicine exactly as prescribed and follow through with your additional treatments such as consuming the correct diet, getting adequate exercise, using stress reduction techniques and so on. Keep your seizure calendar up to date. And don't hesitate to call your doctor if you experience a seizure that's longer or more intense than usual, have any medication-related problems, are given a prescription by another physician, or just have a question.

To Treat or Not to Treat?

A single seizure is usually left untreated because the likelihood of a second seizure occurring is less than 50%. Exposing a patient to potentially harmful side effects simply doesn't make sense when a second seizure might never happen.

However, a single seizure *may* be treated if:

- There is evidence (abnormalities on the EEG or MRI) that a second seizure is likely to happen.

- The initial seizure was lengthy and another prolonged seizure might cause severe complications such as brain damage.

- Other neurological conditions are present such as a stroke, brain tumor or severe head injury.

Once a person has had recurrent epileptic seizures, we typically initiate treatment to prevent the onset of future seizures, especially powerful ones.

But we may not treat a person with epilepsy if:

- They have only simple partial seizures that are not disabling and have no other symptoms. The decision not to treat must be made carefully, however, as there is always a risk that stronger seizures may occur at some point.

- The seizures occur during sleep only and are not typically associated with brain damage. Benign rolandic epilepsy, for example, is characterized by seizures that are restricted to sleep (at least most of the time), and these seizures are outgrown by adolescence.

STEP #2 – AVOID YOUR SEIZURE TRIGGERS

As pointed out in Chapter 2, it's very important to discover your own seizure triggers and take steps to avoid them. Common seizure triggers include:

- sleep deprivation

- traveling across time zones

- hyperventilation (over-breathing)

- emotional stress

- fever or illness

- exposure to flickering lights and different visual screens

- time of the day

- sudden changes in temperature

- hormonal changes

- various medications and supplements (see Appendix 4)

- missed dosages of medication

- alcohol and recreational drugs

For a complete discussion of seizure triggers, see Chapter 2 – What Causes It and Who's At Risk?

STEP #3 – USE THE APPROPRIATE MEDICATIONS

About 70 percent of people with epilepsy patients will gain satisfactory seizure control through medication, although it may take a bit of experimentation before people with the "right" one or the "right" combination of medications is discovered. I cannot stress how important it is to take your medication exactly as directed by your doctor, as even seemingly harmless deviations – such as skipping a dose, forgetting to take them with food (on rare occasions), or taking a generic version instead of the prescribed brand – can lead to serious consequences.

It's also important to be aware that medications are not the sole answer to successful management of epilepsy, since they only suppress seizures. They do not address the mental, emotional, social and legal issues of epilepsy, which may require psychological help, legal assistance, support groups and other services – a comprehensive approach to epilepsy management. However, medications are certainly a cornerstone of treatment.

For a review of the 20-plus medicines used to control seizures, with information on how they are selected and used, common side effects and more, see Chapter 6 – Medications.

STEP #4 –CONSIDER FOLLOWING AN "ANTI-EPILEPSY" DIET

Although there is no such thing as a 100 % proven anti-epilepsy diet, certain people have benefited from following a ketogenic diet, which is high in fat and protein and very low in carbohydrates. The modified Atkins diet and the Low-Glycemic Index diet have also been found to be helpful in controlling epilepsy in some people.

There are also certain foods that should be avoided as they seem to lower the seizure threshold in sensitive people. Chief among these is caffeine (a stimulant), which may lower the threshold directly or indirectly (e.g. by disrupting sleep). Chapter 8 looks at diet therapy for epilepsy.

STEP #5 – ELMINATE THE SEIZURE FOCUS THROUGH SURGERY, IF NECESSARY

Proper diagnosis, avoidance of seizure triggers, taking appropriate medication and eating wisely may be enough for some patients. But for others, these steps will not provide sufficient seizure control. Such patients could benefit from more drastic treatment in the form of surgery.

There are two general approaches to surgery: removing part of the brain, to prevent the genesis or spread of seizures, and implanting a device in the body that delivers an electrical current in order to prevent seizures or stop those already in progress.

All forms of surgery have risks, and the mere thought of operating on the brain is frightening to most people. However, for certain patients, surgery can provide the relief that otherwise eludes them. The surgeries are described in greater detail in Chapter 7.

STEP #6 – EXPLORE SUPPORTIVE, COMPLEMENTARY AND EXPERIMENTAL TREATMENTS

Thus far I've talked about medical therapies that prevent or lessen seizures. But since epilepsy affects nearly every area of your life, it's usually very helpful to explore certain mind/body approaches to health. Psychiatrists and psychologists can help you address emotional issues, and various alternative health practitioners may offer non-traditional approaches to handling the stress and other problems encountered when dealing with epilepsy.

As you'll see in Chapter 9, group therapy or some other form of supportive therapy may help some patients with the handling of emotional problems and lifestyle issues. I also believe that herbs, acupuncture and other forms of alternative therapy should not be discarded as adjuncts to standard treatment, if used under the supervision of a doctor.

AN INTEGRATIVE APPROACH

Rather than attempting to treat seizures with medicines only (the approach taken by many doctors), I advocate a broadly-based treatment and support program. This utilizes the best of standard medicine plus psychological support, diet, alternative medicine and more.

While the six steps described above aren't a one-size-fits-all anti-epilepsy program guaranteed to eliminate seizures forever, they *are* tools that improve epilepsy management and make it possible to live a normal and productive life. And I can say without reservation that, based on my experience, this is *the* best approach to the treatment and management of epilepsy. I've seen it work for thousands of patients, and it can work for you, too.

CHAPTER SIX
MEDICATIONS

Ancient Greeks thought that eating pickled mistletoe might cure epilepsy. Medieval Europeans looked to saints and relics for relief, while Renaissance doctors were likely to prescribe beaver secretions and mugwort. Potassium bromide, the first modern medicine for epilepsy, was developed in the mid 1800s. And today, there are over 20 medications commonly used to treat epileptic seizures in the United States.

These medicines, known collectively as AEDs (antiepileptic drugs), are the mainstay of treatment for epileptic seizures. Typically, AEDs act by suppressing the over-excitation of neurons in the area where the seizures originate, preventing the spread of seizure activity and sometimes stopping it completely. They do this by changing the seizure threshold; that is, "raising the wall" and making it harder for seizures to get started or remain in play. AEDs do not cure epilepsy; they control it. And they can help prevent brain damage and other problems by eliminating certain seizures and reducing the strength of others.

Unfortunately, we do not have a single medicine that works for everyone, as there are many causes and types of seizures and everybody reacts somewhat differently to any given medicine. Thus, about 70 percent of patients are able to control their seizures by taking a single medicine. But for others, two, three or more may be required

– or perhaps no medicine or combination of medicines will prove satisfactory.

It is very important for you to understand which medications are available to treat your seizure type, which ones may be prescribed for you, how they work, how they are metabolized in your body, when you should use them, and when they can safely be discontinued. Then and only then can you be a well-informed member of your treatment team.

WHICH MEDICATION IS RIGHT FOR YOU?

There are many factors that your doctor must consider when choosing a medication for you, including the type of epilepsy you have, your general medical condition, the potential side effects and the cost.

Type of Epilepsy
Some medicines work well for one type of epilepsy but not another. That's one reason it's so important that your diagnosis is correct. This one factor can make the difference between a medication that works and one that either has no effect or worsens the epilepsy.

Side Effects
Each medication has potential side effects, not all of which will pertain to you. (Thank goodness!) Unfortunately, we cannot predict in advance who is going to experience which side effect(s). That's why it's important to inform your doctor immediately if you are experiencing *any* side effects or unusual feelings/occurrences. Most often, he or she will prescribe a different medication that may suit you better. Unfortunately, finding the proper medication can be a process of trial-and-error.

General Medical Condition
It's essential that your doctor compile a complete history of your general health and any other health problems you currently have or have had, and get an accurate list of any medications, herbs or

supplements you're taking. Then, if you happen to have a liver problem, for example, your doctor will know to avoid prescribing any medications that might damage that organ.

Cost of the Medication

It is an unfortunate reality that many patients struggle to afford their medications. There's no advantage to getting prescriptions for the "perfect" medications if you're unable to purchase them. So if cost is an issue, discuss this with your doctor and he or she may prescribe the least expensive medications that will still target your specific problems. Also, there are various programs that can help provide free or low cost medications to those in need. See: http://epilepsylifelinks.com/services_patient-assistance-programs.php for a comprehensive directory of Patient Assistance Programs.

WHAT HAPPENS TO MEDICATIONS IN THE BODY?

Once you take a medication, it is absorbed, enters the bloodstream, is transported to the brain to perform its duties, and is finally eliminated from the body. Let's take a quick look at the absorption, transportation and elimination of medications.

Absorption

The amount of a medicine that is absorbed by the body will vary depending on the route it takes to get into the bloodstream. And that, in turn, depends on how the medicine is formulated and administered:

- **Pill or liquid taken orally** – Only a portion of an AED taken orally will be absorbed, as the digestive system will break down and eliminate some of it. Sometimes, the presence of food either interferes with or aids absorption (depending on the medication), so it's very important to know which medications must be taken with food and which must be taken alone.

It is also important to know which foods should be avoided when taking certain medications.

- **Skin patch** – The absorption rate varies for each medication.

- **Intravenous injection** – The absorption rate is 100%.

- **Intramuscular injection** – The absorption rate is 100%.

- **Rectal suppository** – The absorption rate is close to 100%.

Which route is most effective? That will depend on the medication, your body and the medical condition in question. In other words, it varies, so ask your doctor.

Transportation

Absorption is just the beginning of the medication's journey. It must then travel through the bloodstream to the brain. Some medications move through the bloodstream on their own, while others latch on to carrier proteins via a process called "protein binding." Some AEDs have a high rate of protein binding, which means that much of the medication will be bound to a protein, while a relatively small amount remains "free" and travels on its own. Other AEDs have a low rate or protein binding, with lots of the "free" form in the blood. Others don't bind at all and are completely "free."

Why does this matter? Once the medication arrives at the brain, it will have to pass through the blood-brain barrier, which is designed to keep harmful substances from entering this very critical area. One of the criteria for passing through this barrier is size: only small particles are allowed through. Proteins, however, are not small, which means that any medicine attached to a protein will be excluded. Only "free" medicine will be allowed into the brain. Doctors know how much of any particular medicine is likely to be protein-bound and how much is "free," and calculate the medication dosage accordingly.

Suppose you are taking two medicines with high levels of protein binding, such as Dilantin® and aspirin. Since these two medicines are both very likely to bind to proteins, and there are only a fixed number of proteins in the body, they'll have to compete with each other to latch onto a protein molecule. Some of that Dilantin® is going to "lose" the race and won't find enough protein to latch on to. This means that more Dilantin® than usual will be "free" and pass into the brain. In such a case, the patient could suffer a Dilantin® overdose even when taking a standard amount of the medication! This is just one issue your doctor will have to wrestle with when determining the kind and amount of medication that will be right for you.

Elimination

Almost as soon as a medication arrives on the scene, the body will identify it as a foreign and potentially dangerous substance, and begin to eliminate it. There are two main organs in the body responsible for the elimination of medication: the liver and the kidneys.

- **Liver** – Most, but not all, medicines are transformed by and sometimes inactivated in the liver. This essential process, which helps prevent the build-up of toxic substances in the body, can be upset by the very medicines you're taking to make you healthier. Some medications, called "inducers," make the liver work faster. These include carbamazepine (Tegretol®), phenytoin (Dilantin®) and phenobarbital (Luminal®). Others, such as valproic acid (Depakote®), are "inhibitors" that slow the liver's actions. A medication's ability to make the liver work faster or slower must be taken into account when prescribing medication, for changing the liver's rate of elimination alters the level of the medication in the body.

  For example, when an inducer such as Tegretol® revs up the liver, other medications such as Depakote® will be removed from the body faster than normal. This means that even if you're taking enough Depakote® to keep your seizures under control, adding Tegretol® to the mix could lower your Depakote® levels enough to allow a seizure to occur.

- **Kidneys** – Some medicines, such as levetiracetam (Keppra®) or gabapentin (Neurontin®), are eliminated by the kidneys rather than the liver. If your kidneys are not working well, these medications will accumulate in the body, resulting in significant side effects.

BEFORE TAKING ANY MEDICATION

It's the doctor's job to select the best medicines, but you, the patient, also have an important job: Ask lots of questions to make sure you know exactly how and when the medicine(s) should be taken, how to store them properly, which side effects to watch for, and so on.

General Questions

Ask your doctor the following questions about every medicine prescribed for you, even if you've taken it before.

- Why is this medicine the most beneficial for me?

- What are its potential side effects? Which of these are serious enough to merit a call to you, or a trip to the emergency room?

- Exactly when and how do I take it?

- Can I take it with food?

- How do I store it?

- How soon does it begin to work?

- What should I do if I miss a dose?

- What happens if I take too much, or the levels in my blood rise too high for other reasons?

- What happens if I suddenly stop taking it, or miss a dose?

- Are there are other mediations it interacts with?

- Are there any reasons I should not take it?

Questions Regarding Women's Health

- Does it affect contraceptives?

- Does it affect fertility?

- Is it safe to use during pregnancy?

- Is it safe to use during breastfeeding?

- Will it affect the bones (osteoporosis)?

Questions Regarding Men's Health

- Does it affect sexual performance?

- Does it affect fertility?

Write your questions down *before* you go to your appointment as questions are perishable and have a way of disappearing as soon as the doctor walks into the room!

What About Generic Medications?

There is a great deal of confusion and, at times, heated controversy surrounding generic medications. Are they better/worse than the brand name versions? Are they different in any way? Why is there a cost difference? Before I can answer any of these questions, let's define some terms and go over a few of the basics.

What is a generic medication? A generic medication is a copy of a brand-name medication. The difference is that the brand-name medication is developed, marketed and promoted by a pharmaceutical company. The company receives a patent on the drug for a certain number of years, so they can market the medication exclusively. When that period expires, any manufacturer that follows the FDA guidelines is allowed to produce the drug. The intended use, dosage, administration route, effects and side effects of a generic medication are the same as those seen with the original medication. But because the manufacturers of generics don't have to invest in years of research, development and marketing of these drugs, and because there may be competing versions of the same medications, generics can be much less expensive than brand-name drugs.

How are generics approved? A generic medication must be absorbed, distributed through the body and eliminated in a way that is similar, but not necessarily equal to its brand-name counterpart. And there is where the problem lies. Some generic medications may be absorbed more or less efficiently than the brand-name medication, resulting in drug levels in the body that are not equal to those seen with the brand name. This means that if you switch from a brand name drug to a generic, the amount of medication in your body could suddenly change. If it increases, side effects will be more likely. If it decreases, seizures will be more likely.

Is there only one generic drug for each brand name medication? There could be many companies producing the same medication. Each generic drug will behave a little differently, increasing the potential for side effects or seizures as you move from brand name to generic, or from one generic to another.

Does the same pharmacy provide the same generic medication every time? No. Most pharmacies will buy the generic that happens to be cheaper at any given time. That means that you might be getting a different generic medication each time.

When and how should I use generics? Generics are used when your doctor decides they pose no risk to you, or you cannot afford the brand-name medication. If you are going to use a generic medication, ask your pharmacist if you will be getting the same generic from the same manufacturer every time you refill your prescription. If the pharmacist cannot guarantee this, you may need to choose another pharmacy. Usually, the smaller pharmacies tend to be more accommodating.

How can you tell the difference between generic and brand name medications? The name of a generic typically appears in the lower case form (e.g. acetazolamide), while a brand name is capitalized (e.g. Diamox).

WHEN SHOULD MEDICATION BE STARTED AND STOPPED?

While treating epilepsy with medication is very common, we don't necessarily treat all seizures this way. For example, a single seizure that is not prolonged and is associated with negative test results on EEG, MRI or CT, usually doesn't require medication since the likelihood of a second seizure occurring is less than 50 percent.

And while medication is usually recommended for recurrent epileptic seizures, there are some types that are not treated this way. Benign rolandic epilepsy, for example, produces seizures that occur mainly during sleep, are not associated with brain damage, and are outgrown by adolescence. In this case, medication does not seem to be necessary. Generally, however, usually most recurrent seizures do need to be treated with medication.

Rules for Taking Medication

No matter which medications you may be taking, be sure to follow these rules:

- **Store all medications properly** – Medications should be stored at room temperature (*not* in the refrigerator) and in a low-moisture area (*not* in the bathroom). Be sure to keep them away from children!

- **If you miss a dose, take it as soon as you remember** – If you miss two doses, do *not* take a double dose. Call your doctor immediately.

- **If you take an excessive dose, call your doctor and 911 immediately** -You can also contact the American Association of Poison Control Centers at 1-800-222-1222 for specific information about the medication in question.

- **Do not suddenly stop taking your medication** - Never stop taking your medication without first discussing it with your doctor. Withdrawal of many seizure medications can result in very serious, life-threatening seizures (status epilepticus).

- **If skin rash or difficulty breathing occurs, call your doctor and 911 immediately** - This indicates an allergic reaction and is a MEDICAL EMERGENCY. All medications have the potential to cause allergic reactions, which can be fatal!

Reducing/ Discontinuing Medication

Once I have prescribed a medication for a patient, the first question that many of them ask is, "How long do I have to take this medication? Will I ever be able to stop?"

The answer varies according to the type of epilepsy and the presence/absence of seizures. In most cases, as long as you continue to experience seizures, medication will be required. However, once you have been seizure-free for a certain amount of time (generally 2 to 5 years, as determined by your epileptologist), the dosage can usually be reduced slowly until the medication is discontinued entirely (as long as the seizures do not reappear). In patients who become seizure-free following surgery, medication is usually tapered off after only one year.

Those who experience unacceptable side effects from their medication or prefer to take no medication at all will probably wish to reduce/discontinue AEDs as soon as possible. A typical example is the woman who wants to become pregnant and prefers to be medication-free to avoid potential damage to her baby. But there are also those who may need or want to take medication indefinitely. Certain types of epilepsy (like juvenile myoclonic) are controlled very effectively with medication, but once the medications are stopped, the seizures tend to come back. Those with these kinds of epilepsy may never stop taking their medication. Others may not want to stop their meds because there is an increased risk of recurrent seizures which could lead to trouble on the job or the loss of driving privileges. Whether or not reducing/eliminating your medication is a good idea is a decision that can only be made by you and your epileptologist together

When reducing medication dosages, we doctors always move slowly! Baby steps are taken, unless the medication is producing unacceptable side effects and we need to speed up the process. If this is true in your case, you may need to be admitted to the hospital for a safer withdrawal of medications and constant monitoring.

Depending on your type of epilepsy, there can be a chance that your seizures will recur when your medication is discontinued. With this in mind, be sure to avoid driving or engaging in activities that could put you at risk, especially immediately after reducing or discontinuing your meds, when the risk of recurring seizures is at its highest. Also, be especially careful to avoid seizure triggers such as sleep deprivation, excessive stress and so on.

THE ANTI-EPILEPTIC DRUGS (AEDs)

Now that you know about anti-epileptic drugs in general, which questions to ask before taking medications, the rules for taking medications properly, and when medications are reduced/discontinued, it's time to focus on the anti-epileptic drugs themselves. Over twenty AEDs are used to control seizures, and each has its own mechanism of action, side effect profile and other properties/actions. As it's impossible to discuss every aspect of every AED, I've limited the discussion to key items only. You can find more information about each medicine on my website: www.epilepsygroup.com.

Note: You'll see an unusual-looking "word" – mg/kg/day – in the medication descriptions. It means milligrams of medicine per kilogram of the patient's body weight, per day.

After each medication, in parenthesis, you will find the year in which each medication was approved in the USA.

Adrenocorticotropic Hormone (ACTH)
Brand name(s):
Acthar Gel®

Author's opinion:

ACTH is a powerful hormone created in the body that produces "steroids." Its main use in epilepsy is to treat infantile spasms. As with any powerful medication, it has potential serious side effects which should be monitored closely and will require that you work very closely with your doctor. In spite of these potential problems, ACTH may significantly improve seizure control and brain development in patients with infantile spasms.

Type of epilepsy it helps:

ACTH is mainly used for infantile spasms.

Method of administration:

Injection

Average dose:

There is no agreement as to the correct dose of ACTH for infantile spasms. Dose and the duration of treatment (which could range from a few to several weeks) will vary according to the treating epilepsy center.

How long before it produces a steady effect?

Usually during the first one to two weeks of treatment.

Blood work needed:

It is necessary to check blood sugar.

Possible side effects:

- Cardiac: enlargement of the heart (usually resolves once treatment is stopped), high blood pressure
- Eyes: cataracts, glaucoma
- GI: gastric ulcers
- Psychiatric: behavioral and mood changes

- Systemic: worsening of diabetes, increased risk of infections, weight gain

Close monitoring for side effects is always required during ACTH treatment.

Other AEDs that can increase the blood level of ACTH:
None anticipated

Other AEDs that can decrease the blood level of ACTH:
None anticipated

Other drug interactions:
None anticipated

Who should *not* take this medication?
Do not take this medication if you have severe hypertension, diabetes, gastric ulcers, low immunity and allergic reaction to this medication.

Acetazolamide (1953)
Brand name(s):
Diamox®

Author's opinion:
This medication is a mild diuretic ("water pill") and a weak anticonvulsant. I use it mainly in women whose seizures are related to their menstrual cycles (catamenial epilepsy). Even though there are not many studies confirming the anticonvulsant effect, I have observed good results.

An often welcome side effect is a diminished appetite, which promotes weight loss. This effect could be useful when combined with medications that tend to increase appetite/weight gain like valproic acid (Depakote®).

Type of epilepsy it helps:
Partial and generalized epilepsy, related to menstrual cycles.

Other uses:
Acetazolamide is a mild diuretic

Method of administration:
Capsule, extended-release capsule or tablet, usually taken 2-3 times per day, with or without food.

Average dose:
- Adults: 8 to 16 mg/kg (in divided doses) with an optimum range of 375-1000 mg/day. It is usually started slowly.

How long before it produces a steady effect?
Unknown

Blood work needed:
No

Possible side effects:
- Decreased potassium levels
- Loss of appetite and weight, changes in taste
- Abnormal sensations and tingling, mainly around the mouth

Other AEDs that can increase the blood level of acetazolamide:
None anticipated

Other AEDs that can decrease the blood level of acetazolamide:
None anticipated

Other drug interactions:
- Increases levels of carbamazepine (Tegretol®, Carbatrol®), phenobabrbital (Luminal®) and phenytoin (Dilantin®) levels.
- Decreases levels of primidone (Mysoline®).

Who should *not* take this medication?

Do not take this medication if you have:
- Allergies to this medication or any sulfa drugs (includes many antibiotics and seizure medications like topiramate and zonisamide)
- Low blood levels of sodium or potassium
- Kidney or liver disease

Carbamazepine (1974)

Brand name(s):

Tegretol®, Tegretol XR®, Carbatrol®

Author's opinion:

Carbamazepine is an excellent first-line medication for partial epilepsy. Since it can make generalized epilepsy worse, an accurate diagnosis is very important. Carbamazepine may produce certain side effects depending on the amount taken, so it must be started slowly. Allergic reactions are rare but can be serious. Blood work should be done periodically to monitor for potential side effects.

Type of epilepsy it helps:

Partial epilepsy. It may make generalized epilepsy worse (mainly absence and myoclonic seizures).

Other uses:

Because carbamazepine has a mood stabilizing effect, it is sometimes used in bipolar disorder. It is also used for certain kinds of pain.

Method of administration:

In capsule, tablet or oral suspension form, carbamazepine is taken 2 to 4 times a day with food. There is an extended-release formula that is taken 2 times a day with or without food.

Note: You may notice the coating of the extended-release tablet in your stool. Do not panic! It is the coating that allows the medication to be released slowly.

Average dose:
- Children: Dose is based on age.
- Adults: 400-1200 mg/day, 3 or 4 times a day but it is tapered up slowly and started at a low dose.

How long before it produces a steady effect?
2-3 days, but may take up to 2 weeks for levels to become stable. Carbamazepine induces the liver to work more, resulting in eliminating itself faster. This process is usually completed by 3-5 weeks after fixed dosing regimen of Carbamazepine. Levels of this medication therefore may decrease and the dose of medication may need to be increased.

Blood work needed:
Blood work is recommended more frequently at the beginning of treatment (monthly) Later, it can be done every 4-6 months to monitor blood cells, liver function and sodium levels, among other things. Monitoring blood levels of medication can help to guide treatment.

Possible side effects:
High doses of carbamazepine may produce:
- Blurred or double vision
- Drowsiness, fatigue
- Lack of coordination (clumsiness)
- Decreased sodium levels in the blood, which can lead to sleepiness, an increase in seizures and coma

These side effects are usually reversed by decreasing the dose.
Other side effects include:
- Allergic reactions

- Blood cell changes, including a decrease in red cells, white cells and platelets known as *aplastic anemia*. In this case, the medication must be stopped immediately (after consultation with your doctor).
- Chest pain, which indicates cardiac problems and is a MEDICAL EMERGENCY that you must report to your doctor immediately.
- Decreased effectiveness of contraceptives.
- Depression that may lead to suicidal thoughts/behavior. This is a MEDICAL EMERGENCY. Report depression to your doctor immediately.
- Decrease in blood levels of sodium, which could lead to an increase in sleepiness, seizures and risk of coma.
- GI symptoms such as liver problems, nausea, vomiting, abdominal pain, and dryness of the mouth
- Osteoporosis, caused by depletion of vitamin D and calcium.

Medications that increase the blood level of carbamazepine:

If any of these medications are used in addition to carbamazepine, toxic side effects may occur:

- AEDs: felbamate (Felbatol®), and valproic acid (Depakote®)
- Antacid medications: cimetidine (Tagamet®)
- Antibiotics: chloramphenicol, clarithromycin (Biaxin®), doxycycline, (Vibramycin®), erythromycin (E-Mycin®), isoniazid (Tubizid®), metronidazole (Flagyl®), and troleandromycin (Flexyx®)
- Antidepressants: amitryptiline (Elavil®), doxepin (Sinequan®), fluoxetine (Prozac®), fluvoxamine (Luvox®), nefazadone (Serzone®), nortryptiline (Pamelor®) and voloxazine (Vivalan®)
- Antifungals: ketoconazole (Nizoral®)
- Blood thinners: ticlopidine (Ticlid®)
- Calcium channel blockers (heart medications): such as diltiazem (Cartia®), nifedipine (Adalat®), verapamil (Calan®)

- Major psychiatric medications: haloperidol (Haldol®)
- Pain medications: propoxyphene (Darvon®)

In addition, grapefruit juice increases carbamazepine levels.

Other medications/herbs that decrease the blood level of carbamazepine:
- AEDs: phenobarbital (Luminal®), phenytoin (Dilantin®), primidone (Mysoline®), oxcarbazepine (Trileptal®), zonisamide (Zonegran®)
- Herbs: St. John's Wort

Carbamazepine's effects on other important medications:
Carbamazepine reduces levels of:
- AEDs: clobazam (Frisium®), clonazepam (Klonopin®), diazepam (Valium®), ethosuximide (Zarontin®), felbamate (Felbatol®), lamotrigine (Lamictal®), phenobarbital (Luminal®), primidone (Mysoline®), topiramate (Topamax®), valproic acid (Depakote®), zonisamide (Zonergan®)
- Blood thinners: warfarin (Coumadin®)
- Immunosuppressants: cyclosporin A (Gengraf®)
- Oral contraceptives
- Tricyclic antidepressants: amitriptyline (Elavil®)

Who should *not* take this medication?
Do not take carbamazepine if you:
- Are allergic to carbamazepine or oxcarbazepine
- Are currently taking (or have taken in the past two weeks) medications used for depression called "MAO inhibitors" (marplan®, nardil®, eldepryl® and parnate®)
- Have a history of bone marrow suppression
- Have had positive genetic testing for HLA-B*1502**

**If you have had positive genetic testing for HLA-B*1502, you are at risk of severe allergic skin reactions when taking this medication. Asian patients are more likely to carry this genetic variation and should be tested before starting carbamazepine.

Ethosuximide (1960)
Brand name(s):
Zarontin®

Author's opinion:
Ethosuximide is a first-line medication used exclusively for absence seizures. Overall it is very safe, but some blood work needs to be done periodically to monitor for side effects.

Type of epilepsy it helps:
Absence epilepsy

Method of administration:
Capsule and syrup (raspberry-flavored). Due to frequent GI discomfort, it is recommended that ethosuximide be taken with food.

Average dose:
- Children: age 3-6, 250 mg/day; age 6+, 500mg/day (Average dose: = 20mg/kg/day)
- Adults: 20 mg/kg/day
- It is started slowly to avoid side effects

How long before it produces a steady effect?
4-10 days

Blood work needed:
Blood work is recommended every 4-6 months to monitor blood cells and liver function, among others. Monitoring blood levels of medication can help to guide treatment.

Possible side effects:

- GI: upset stomach, nausea, vomiting, abdominal pain and diarrhea
- Other: Fatigue, drowsiness, headache, dizziness, hiccups, depression, nervousness, irritability and night terrors

Serious side effects:

- Allergic reactions

Other AEDs that may increase the blood level of ethosuximide:

Valproic acid (Depakote®) will increase it slightly.

Other AEDs that may decrease the blood level of ethosuximide:

Carbamazepine (Tegretol®, Carbatrol®), phenobarbital (Luminal®), phenytoin (Dilantin®) and primidone (Mysoline®).

Other drug interactions:

- Antibiotics: Rifampin (Rifadin®) will decrease levels of ethosuximide
- Antituberculars: Isoniazid (Niazid®) will increase levels of ethosuximide.

Who should *not* take this medication?

Do not take ethosuximide if you are allergic to it.

Felbamate (1993)
Brand name(s):

Felbatol®

Author's opinion:

Felbamate is a powerful and effective medication; however, due to very serious side effects, it should only be used when all other medications have failed. Patients must be closely monitored due to a high risk of developing aplastic anemia and liver toxicity. (Felbamate was taken off the market, then brought back with severe warnings in 1994.)

Type of epilepsy it helps:

Partial and generalized, in particular Lennox-Gastaut syndrome. Due to its serious side effects, felbamate is only used for very difficult to control seizures

Method of administration:

Tablet and oral suspension, taken 3-4 times per day, with or without food.

Average dose:
- Children: Initial dose is 15 mg/kg/day (in divided doses); may be increased up to 20-45 mg/kg/day
- Adults: Initial dose is 1200 mg/day (in divided doses); may be increased in 600 mg increments every 2 weeks to 3600 mg/day

How long before it produces a steady effect?

Two to five days

Blood work needed:

Blood work is initially recommended more frequently (every 2-4 weeks) and after being on this medication for longer time periodically (every 3-6 months) to check blood cells and liver function. Blood tests need to be performed for significant amount of time after discontinuation of medication.

Possible side effects:
- GI: upset stomach, vomiting, constipation, diarrhea and decreased appetite.

- Other: insomnia, headache, anxiety, blurred vision, fatigue, weight loss and facial swelling.

Serious side effects:
- Acute liver failure (1 in 24,000 to 34,000),
- Allergic reactions
- Anemia (severe) - may be fatal (1 in 3,600 to 5,000)
- Risk of suicidal thoughts and behavior

Other AEDs that can increase the blood level of felbamate:

Valproic acid (Depakote®)

Other AEDs that can decrease the blood level of felbamate:

Phenobarbital (Luminal®), phenytoin (Dilantin®), primidone (Mysoline®), carbamazepine (Tegretol®, Carbatrol®)

Other drug interactions:

Felbamate increases levels of:
- AEDS: carbamazepine (Tegretol®, Carbatrol®) toxic metabolite, phenobarbital (Luminal®), phenytoin (Dilantin®), and valproic acid (Depakote®).
- Blood thinners: warfarin (Coumadin®)

Felbamate decreases levels of:
- Oral contraceptives: May render them less effective, resulting in unintended pregnancy.

Who should *not* take this medication?

Do not take felbamate if you have liver disease, abnormal conditions of the blood or are allergic to this medication.

Gabapentin (1993)
Brand name(s):

Neurontin®

Author's opinion:

This is a weak anticonvulsant with minimal side effects and almost no interactions with other medications. While gabapentin is almost ideal from the side effects point of view, it rarely helps to control seizures.

Type of epilepsy it helps:

Partial epilepsy

Other uses:

Pain and restless leg syndrome

Method of administration:

Tablet, capsules and oral solution, taken by mouth with or without food, 3 times a day.

Average dose:
- Children: Initial dose is 10-15 mg/kg/day (divided three times a day); 40 mg/kg/day (divided three times a day) for children 3-4 years; 25-35 mg/kg/day (divided three times a day) for those 5 and up.
- Adults: Initial dose is 300 mg (divided three times a day); then may be increased up to 1800 mg/day

How long before it produces a steady effect?

1-2 days

Blood work needed:

Baseline only to check kidney function among others.

Possible side effects:
- GI: upset stomach, constipation, increased appetite, weight gain

- Other: drowsiness, dizziness, difficulty with coordination, impaired memory, twitching, excessive emotional reactions, nervousness, depression, swelling of the feet.

Serious side effects:
- Allergic reactions
- Risk of suicidal thoughts and behavior

Other AEDs that can increase the blood level of gabapentin:
None anticipated

Other AEDs that can decrease the blood level of gabapentin:
None anticipated

Other drug interactions:
Antacids can slightly reduce the level of gabapentin.

Who should *not* take this medication?
Do not take gabapentin if you are allergic to this medication or have kidney failure (as it is eliminated through the kidneys).

Lacosamide (2008)
Brand name(s):
Vimpat ®

Authors's opinion:
Lacosamide is a very effective medication for partial epilepsy with few reported side effects. As it is a fairly new medication, side effects may become more evident over time.

Type of epilepsy it helps:
Partial epilepsy

Method of administration:
Tablet, oral solution, and injection, taken twice a day with or without food.

Average dose:

Initial dose is 50 mg (divided twice a day); recommended maintenance dose 200-400 mg/day (in divided doses), although higher doses are sometimes used.

How long before it produces a steady effect?

3 days

Blood work needed:

Blood work is recommended every 4-6 months to monitor blood cells and liver function, among others.

Possible side effects:
- Brain: dizziness, headaches, double vision, fatigue, lack of coordination
- Cardiac: irregular heartbeat (very rarely)
- GI: nausea, liver toxicity

Serious side effects:
- Allergic reactions
- Increased risk of suicidal thoughts or behavior

Other AEDs that can increase the blood level of lacosamide:

None anticipated

Other AEDs that can decrease the blood level of lacosamide:
None anticipated

Other drug interactions:

None anticipated.

Who should *not* take this medication?

Do not take lacosamide if you are allergic to this medication, have liver problems or have prolonged PR intervals in the EKG (a cardiologic problem).

Lamotrigine (1994)
Brand name(s):

Lamictal®

Author's opinion:

This is a first-line, very effective medication that works well for partial and generalized epilepsy. Lamotrigine needs to be started slowly, which means it can't be used for emergencies. It produces almost no cognitive side effects and is usually very well tolerated. Skin rash could be very serious, so this needs to be monitored closely, especially when the medication is first taken.

Type of epilepsy it helps:

Partial and generalized epilepsy (including Lennox-Gastaut syndrome)

Other uses:

Bipolar disorder, as it is a mood stabilizer

Method of administration:

Regular, chewable or extended-release tablets. In order to minimize the chances of side effects and skin rash, lamotrigine must be started very slowly, especially if taken in conjunction with valproic acid (Depakote®).

Average dose:
- Children: Initial dose is 0.3 mg/kg/day (in divided doses); maintenance dose is 4.5-7.5 mg/kg/day (in divided doses). Dosage will be different for those also taking other seizure medications, especially valproic acid (Depakote®).
- Adults: Initial dose is 25 mg/day; maintenance dose is100-400 mg/day (in divided doses). Dosage will be different for those also taking other seizure medications, especially valproic acid (Depakote®).

How long before it produces a steady effect?

5 days

Blood work needed:

Blood work is recommended every 4-6 months to monitor blood cells and liver function, among others. Monitoring blood levels of medication can help to guide treatment.

Possible side effects:

- GI: nausea, vomiting, diarrhea, upset stomach, constipation and liver toxicity
- Skin: rash and itching
- Other: dizziness, insomnia and headache

Note: Lamotrigine usually has a positive effect on mood.

Serious side effects:

- Serious skin rash, including Stevens-Johnson syndrome
- Lamotrigine may cause suicidal thoughts or actions in a very small number of people.
- Aseptic meningitis (inflammation of the membrane that covers the brain and spinal cord). Presenting symptoms are: headache, fever, nausea, vomiting, stiff neck, rash, unusual sensitivity to light, muscle pains, chills, confusion, or drowsiness.

Other AEDs that can increase the blood level of lamotrigine:

Valproic acid (Depakote®)

Other AEDs that can decrease the blood level of lamotrigine:

Carbamazepine (Tegretol®, Carbatrol®), oxcarbazepine (Trileptal®), phenobarbital (Luminal®), phenytoin (Dilantin®), primidone (Mysoline®) and topiramate (Topamax®).

Other drug interactions:

- Could decrease levels of valproic acid (Depakote®).
- Lamotrigine levels are lowered by the estrogen in birth control pills or hormone replacement therapy, the antibiotic rifampin (Rifadin®), and acetaminophen (Tylenol®).
- Lamotrigine levels are increased by the antidepressant sertraline (Zoloft®).

Who should *not* take this medication?

Do not take lamotrigine if you have severe myoclonic epilepsy or are allergic to this medication.

Levetiracetam (1999)
Brand name(s):

Keppra®

Author's opinion:

Levetiracetam is a first-line, very effective medication that can be started at high doses with minimal side effects: overall it is an excellent medication. Because it is not metabolized through the liver, levetiracetam cannot cause liver damage. In some cases, mainly in children, irritability and behavioral changes are seen, limiting its use. Vitamin B6 may help ease these behavioral changes.

Type of epilepsy it helps:

Generalized and partial epilepsy

Method of administration:

As a tablet, oral solution or injection, levetiracetam is taken twice a day with or without food. Extended-release formulations are taken once a day.

Average dose:

- Children: Initial dose is 10 mg/kg (divided; twice a day); then increased to 60 mg/kg (divided; twice a day)

- Adults: Initial dose is 500 mg (divided; twice a day), then increased to as much as 3000 mg (divided; twice a day)

How long before it produces a steady effect?
2-3 days

Blood work needed:
Blood work is recommended at baseline to monitor blood cells and kidney function. Liver function tests are not necessary as this medication is not eliminated through the liver

Possible side effects:
- Brain: drowsiness, dizziness, difficulty with coordination, memory problems, headache, depression, nervousness, anxiety and hostility.

Serious side effects:
- Increased risk of suicidal thoughts or behavior

Other AEDs that can increase the blood level of levetiracetam:
None anticipated

Other AEDs that can decrease the blood level of levetiracetam:
None anticipated

Other drug interactions:
None anticipated

Who should *not* take this medication?
Do not take if you have:
- Allergies to this medication
- Kidney malfunction (levetiracetam is eliminated through the kidneys)

Oxcarbazepine (2000)
Brand name(s):

Trileptal®

Author's opinion:

Oxcarbazepine, which is very similar to carbamazepine, is a first-line medication used for partial epilepsy. It must be started slowly to avoid side effects, but is usually very well tolerated. Blood sodium levels must be monitored periodically, mainly in older patients.

Type of epilepsy it helps:

Partial epilepsy

Method of administration:

Tablet or oral suspension, taken twice daily with or without food.

Average dose:
- Children: Initial dose is 8-10 mg/kg/day (divided; twice a day), then increased to an Average dose: of 31 mg/kg/day
- Adults: Initial dose is 300 mg/day (divided; twice a day), then increased to 1200 mg/day (divided; twice a day)

How long before it produces a steady effect?

2-3 days

Blood work needed:

Blood work is recommended more frequently (monthly) at the beginning of treatment. Then it may be done every 4-6 months to monitor blood cells, liver function and sodium levels, among others. Monitoring blood levels of medication can help to guide treatment.

Possible side effects:
- GI: nausea, vomiting, abdominal pain, diarrhea and constipation

- Other: dizziness, drowsiness, difficulty with coordination, fatigue, blurry or double vision, and decreased sodium levels in the blood. Most of these side effects can be reduced or eliminated by reducing the dose.

Serious side effects:
- Allergic reactions
- Risk of suicidal thoughts or behavior
- Very low sodium levels in the blood.

Other AEDs that can increase the blood level of oxcarbazepine:
None anticipated

Other AEDs that can decrease the blood level of oxcarbazepine:
Carbamazepine (Tegretol®, Carbatrol®), phenobarbital (Luminal®) and phenytoin (Dilantin®)

Other drug interactions:
Oxcarbazepine reduces:
- Efficacy of oral contraceptives
- Levels of lamotrigine (Lamictal®) in the blood

Who should *not* take this medication?
Do not take if you have:
- Allergies to this medication or to carbamazepine (Tegretol®, Carbatrol®).
- Liver disease
- Low sodium levels in the blood

Phenobarbital (1910)
Brand name(s):
Luminal®

Author's opinion:

One of the oldest medications used for seizures, phenobarbital is very effective and quite inexpensive. However, its use is limited due to cognitive side effects.

Type of epilepsy it helps:

Partial epilepsy and generalized tonic-clonic seizures

Method of administration:

As a tablet, oral suspension or injection, phenobarbital can be taken 1 to 3 times per day with or without food.

Average dose:

- Children: 4-8 mg/kg/day (in divided doses).
- Adults: 60 mg/day (increased gradually to a target dose of 90-120 mg/day or higher)

How long does it take to start having a steady effect?

2-3 weeks

Blood work needed:

Blood work is recommended every 4-6 months to monitor blood cells and liver function, among others. Monitoring blood levels of medication can help to guide treatment.

Possible side effects:

- Brain: sedation, drowsiness, fatigue, dizziness and headache. In children, it may cause hyperactivity.
- GI: nausea, vomiting and liver toxicity
- Skin: scaling of the skin
- Other: anemia, osteoporosis, sexual dysfunction and shallow breathing

Serious side effects:

- Allergic reactions
- Dependence
- Risk of suicidal thoughts or behavior

Other AEDs that may increase the blood level of phenobarbital:

Felbamate (Felbatol®) and valproic acid (Depakote®)

Other AEDs that may decrease the blood level of phenobarbital:

None anticipated.

Other drug interactions:

Phenobarbital lowers levels of:

- AEDs: carbamazepine (Tegretol®, Carbatrol®), clobazam (Frisium®), clonazepam (Klonopin®), diazepam (Valium®), etosuximide (Zarontin®),felbamate (Felbatol®), lamotrigine (Lamictal®), lorazepam (Ativan®), tiagabine (Gabitril®), topiramate (Topamax®), valproic acid (Depakote®) and zonisamide (Zonegran®),
- Antidepressants: tricyclics (Elavil®) and SSRI paroxetine (Paxil®)
- Blood thinners: warfarin (Coumadin®)
- Cardiac medications: digoxin (Lanoxin®)
- Hormones: estrogen and steroids

These medications/supplements decrease phenobarbital levels:

- Antibiotics: chloramphenicol
- Supplements: folate and vitamin B6

These medications increase phenobarbital levels:

- Antibiotics: isoniazid (Niazid®)
- Antimalarials: quinine (Qualaquin®)

Who should *not* take this medication?

Do not take if you have:
- Acute intermittent porphyria
- Allergies to phenobarbital or the class of drugs called barbiturates
- Liver problems
- Respiratory disease

Phenytoin (1938)
Brand name(s):
Dilantin®, Phenytek®

Author's opinion:

Phenytoin is a first-line, very effective medication for partial epilepsy that can also help generalized tonic-clonic seizures. However, it may make absence and myoclonic seizures worse, making it very important that the epilepsy diagnosis be accurate. While inexpensive, phenytoin has many potential side effects that limit its use.

Type of epilepsy it helps:

Partial epilepsy

Method of administration:

As a capsule, extended-release capsule, chewable tablet, oral suspension or injection, phenytoin is taken 1-3 times daily with or without food. Some antacids will impair its absorption.

Average dose:
- Children: 4-10 mg/kg/day (may be divided doses, taken two or three times a day). Close monitoring of blood levels is especially recommended in infants.
- Adults: 300 mg once a day, although twice a day is necessary for some people.

How long does it take to start having a steady effect?

5-10 days

Blood work needed:

Blood work is recommended every 4-6 months to monitor blood cells and liver function, among others. Monitoring blood levels of medication can help to guide treatment.

Possible side effects:

- Blood: low platelet count, decrease in white cells and red cells
- Brain: impaired coordination, slurred speech, confusion, double vision, which usually occur when taking high doses of the medication and can be reversed by lowering the dose. Long- term use of phenytoin may cause damage to the cerebellum (the part of the brain responsible for coordination).
- Cosmetic: coarsening of the facial features, facial hair growth, enlargement of the lips, swelling and bleeding of the gums
- GI: nausea, vomiting, constipation and potential liver damage.
- Other: Rash, redness, itching, burning, osteoporosis (over the long term) and neuropathy (damage to the nerves affecting the hands and feet).

Serious side effects:

- Allergic skin rash (severe)
- Blood cell problems (severe)
- Liver damage (severe)
- Lymphoma
- Risk of suicidal thoughts or behavior

Other AEDs that may increase the blood level of phenytoin:

Valproic acid (Depakote®), topiramate (Topamax®), felbamate (Felbatol®)

Other AEDs that may decrease the blood level of phenytoin:

Phenobarbital (Luminal®), primidone (Mysoline®), carbamazepine (Tegretol®, Carbatrol®)

Other drug interactions:

Phenytoin will lower levels of:

- AEDs: carbamazepine (Tegretol®, Carbatrol®), clonazepam (Klonopin®), diazepam (Valium®), etosuximide (Zarontin®), felbamate (Felbatol®), lamotrigine (Lamictal®), lorazepam (Ativan®), tiagabine (Gabitril®), topiramate (Topamax®), valproic acid (Depakote®) and zonisamide (Zonegran®)
- Antibiotics: rifampin (Rifadin®), ciprofloxacin (Cipro®) and doxycycline (Vibramycin®)
- Blood thinners: warfarin (Coumadin®)
- Cardiac medications: amiodarone (Cardarone®)
- Hormones: estrogens and steroids and contraceptives.
- Vitamin D

These medications increase phenytoin levels:

- Antacids: cimetidine (Tagamet®)
- Antibiotics: chloramphenicol (Chloromycetin®), isoniazid (Tubizid®), metronidazole (Flagyl®), sulfonamides (Bactrim®, etc)
- Antidepressants: fluoxetine (Prozac®), sertraline (Zoloft®)
- Antifungals: fluconazol (Diflucan®), itraconazole (Sporanox®)
- Blood thinners: ticlopidine (Ticlid®)
- Disulfiram (Antabuse®)
- Pain medications: propoxyphere (Darvon®)

Who should *not* take this medication?

Do not take if you have:

- Acute intermittent porphyria

- Allergies to phenytoin
- Generalized epilepsy (any form), as it may worsen absence and myoclonic seizures
- Liver disease or a history of liver disease

Pregabalin (2004)
Brand name(s):
Lyrica®

Author's opinion:
Pregabalin is a mild seizure medication that has minimal interactions with other medications.

Type of epilepsy it helps:
Partial epilepsy

Other uses:
Pain, fibromyalgia and anxiety

Method of administration:
Pregabalin is taken as a capsule or oral solution 2-3 times per day, with or without food.

Average dose:
- Adults: 150-600 mg/day (divided; twice a day or three times a day)

How long before it produces a steady effect?
1-2 days

Blood work needed:
Blood work is done at baseline to monitor kidney function among others. There is no need to check liver function.

Possible side effects:
- Brain: dizziness, drowsiness, impaired coordination, tremors, memory problems, difficulty with speech, twitching, confusion, blurred vision
- GI: Increased appetite, nausea, gas, bloating, constipation

Serious side effects:
- Allergic reactions (severe)
- Swelling of the throat, head and neck
- Risk of suicidal thoughts or behavior

Other AEDs that can increase the blood level of pregabalin:
None anticipated

Other AEDs that can decrease the blood level of pregabalin:
None anticipated

Other drug interactions:
None anticipated

Who should *not* take this medication?
Do not take pregabalin if you have:
- Allergies to this medication
- Kidney failure (as this medication is eliminated through the kidneys)

Primidone (1954)
Brand name(s):
Mysoline®

Author's opinion:
Primidone breaks down into phenobarbital in the body and, therefore, shares many of the same characteristics. Even though it is

an effective medication, primidone's use is limited due to its sedative properties.

Type of epilepsy it helps:

Partial epilepsy

Method of administration:

Tablet and is taken 3-4 times a day, with or without food.

Average dose:

- Children: 125-250 mg (taken 3 times a day) or approximately 10-25 mg/kg/day
- Adults: 125-250 mg (taken 3 or 4 times a day) or approximately 20 mg/kg/day

How long before it produces a steady effect?

3-10 days

Blood work needed:

Blood work is recommended every 4-6 months to monitor blood cells and liver function among others. Monitoring blood levels of medication can help to guide treatment.

Possible side effects:

- Brain: Drowsiness, hyperirritability, emotional disturbances, anxiety, depression, fatigue, and difficulty with coordination

Serious side effects:

- Allergic reactions
- Risk of suicidal thoughts or behavior.

Other AEDs that may increase the blood level of primidone:

Valproic acid (Depakote®)

Other AEDs that may decrease the blood level of primidone:

None anticipated.

Other drug interactions:

Primidone (via its metabolite phenobarbital) will lower levels of:

- AEDs: carbamazepine (Tegretol® and Carbatrol®), di-azepam (Valium®), felbamate (Felbatol®), lamotrigine (Lamictal®), lorazepam (Ativan®), tiagabine (Gabitril®), topiramate (Topamax®), valproic acid (Depakote®) and zonisamide (Zonegran®).
- Blood thinners: warfarin (Coumadin®).
- Hormones: estrogen and steroids

Note: Isonazid (Niazid®) inhibits the conversion of primidone to phenobarbital and may cause side effects such as sleepiness and fatigue due to an accumulation of primidone.

Who should *not* take this medication?

Do not take primidone if you have:

- Acute intermittent porphyria
- Allergies to primidone or phenobarbital

Rufinamide (2008)
Brand name(s):

Banzel®

Author's opinion:

Rufinamide is a new medication specifically used for Lennox-Gastaut syndrome. I have observed very good results with this medication, with minimal side effects.

Type of epilepsy it helps:

Lennox-Gastaut syndrome

Method of administration:

Tablet and oral suspension taken twice a day. Rufinamide should be taken with food, as it improves absorption of the medication.

Average dose:

- Children: Initial dose of 10 mg/kg/day (in divided doses), increasing to a target dose of 45 mg/kg/day (in divided doses)
- Adults: Initial dose of 400-800 mg/day (in divided doses), increasing to a maximum dose of 3200 mg/day (in divided doses)

How long before it produces a steady effect?

2 days

Blood work needed:

Periodic (4-6 months) blood work is recommended to check blood cells and liver function among others.

Possible side effects:

- Brain: drowsiness, headache, fatigue, dizziness, impaired coordination, attention problems and aggression
- GI: vomiting, nausea, decreased appetite and abdominal pain.
- Other: rash, itching and decrease in white blood cells.

Serious side effects:

- Risk of suicidal thoughts or behavior.

Other AEDs that can increase the blood level of rufinamide:

- Valproic acid (Depakote®)

Other AEDs that can decrease the blood level of rufinamide:

Carbamazepine (Tegretol®. Carbatrol®), phenobarbital (Luminal®), phenytoin (Dilantin®), and primidone (Mysoline®)

Other drug interactions:

Rufinamide may decrease the effectiveness of hormonal contraceptives.

Who should *not* take this medication?

Do not take rufinamide if you have:
- Allergies to this medication.
- Familial Short QT syndrome (a very rare heart condition)

Tiagabine (1997)
Brand name(s):

Gabitril®

Author's opinion:

Tiagabine is a mild seizure medication, not used as first-line.

Type of epilepsy it helps:

Partial

Method of administration:

Tablet, taken 2-4 times a day with food.

Average dose:

Initial dose is 4 mg/day to maximum dose of 32 to 56 mg (divided; twice a day or four times a day)

How long before it produces a steady effect?

2 days

Blood work needed:

Periodic (4-6 months) blood work is recommended to check blood cells and liver function among others.

Possible side effects:
- Brain: dizziness, drowsiness, tremor, difficulty with concentration/attention, insomnia, impaired coordination, confusion and mood changes
- GI: nausea, diarrhea, vomiting and increased appetite

Serious side effects:
- Status epilepticus
- Risk of suicidal thoughts or behavior.

Other AEDs that can increase the blood level of tiagabine:
None anticipated

Other AEDs that can decrease the blood level of tiagabine:
Carbamazepine (Tegretol®, Carbatrol®), phenobarbital (Luminal®), phenytoin (Dilantin®) and primidone (Mysoline®)

Other drug interactions:
None anticipated

Who should *not* take this medication?
Do not take tiagabine if you have:
- Allergies to this medication
- Primary generalized epilepsy, especially absence or myoclonic seizure types, as it can severely worsen it

Topiramate (1996)
Brand name(s):
Topamax®

Author's opinion:
Topiramate is a first-line medication for seizures. However, some patients experience significant cognitive side effects that limit its use.

Types of epilepsy it helps:
Partial and generalized; also used for infantile spasms and Lennox-Gastaut syndrome

Other uses:
Migraine prevention

Method of administration:

Capsule and tablet, taken twice daily with or without food.

Average dose:

- Children: Initial dose is 1-3 mg/kg/day, increasing to a total daily dose of 5-9 mg/kg/day. Higher doses may be needed when combined with other seizure medications.
- Adults: Initial dose is 25-50 mg/day (in divided doses), increasing to a total daily dose 100-200 mg/day (in divided doses). Higher doses may be required when used in combination with other seizure medications.

How long before it produces a steady effect?

4 days

Blood work needed:

Blood work is recommended every 4-6 months to monitor blood cells and liver function, among others. Monitoring blood levels of medication can help to guide treatment.

Possible side effects:

- Brain: dizziness, lack of coordination, drowsiness, insomnia, difficulty concentrating, confusion, cognitive problems, mood problems, depression and anxiety
- GI: diarrhea, constipation, abdominal pain, acid reflux, anorexia, weight loss with potential liver damage.

Serious side effects:

- Decreased sweating which could lead to overheating,
- Impaired vision, eye pain, glaucoma
- Kidney stones
- Risk of suicidal thoughts or behavior

Other AEDs that can increase the blood level of topiramate:

None anticipated

Other AEDs that can decrease the blood level of topiramate:

Carbamazepine (Tegretol® and Carbatrol®), phenobarbital (Luminal®), phenytoin (Dilantin®) and primidone (Mysoline®)

Other drug interactions:

Topiramate decreases the levels of:
- AEDs: valproic acid (Depakote®)
- Cardiac: digoxin (Lanoxin®)

Topiramate reduces efficacy of:

- Oral contraceptves, when topiramate is taken in doses of greater than 200 mg per day.

Topiramate increases levels of:
- Phenytoin (Dilantin®)

Who should *not* take this medication?
Do not take topiramate if you are allergic to this medication.

Vigabatrin (2009)
Brand name(s):

Sabril®

Author's opinion:

Vigabatrin is a powerful medication, mainly prescribed for patients with infantile spasms, especially those who have tuberous sclerosis. However, permanent loss (starting at periphery of visual field) of vision occurs frequently, severely limiting the use of this medication.

Type of epilepsy it helps:

Partial epilepsy, as well as infantile spasms (mainly those with tuberous sclerosis)

Method of administration:

Tablet

Average dose:
- Children: 150 mg/kg, divided; twice a day
- Adults: Initial dose is 2-3 g/day (divided; twice a day), up to 3-4 g/ divided; twice a day

How long before it produces a steady effect?

2 days

Blood work needed:

Baseline blood work is done to measure kidney function among others.

Possible side effects:
- Brain: headache, drowsiness, dizziness, memory impairment, disturbance in attention, sedation, difficulty with speech, irritability, depression, confusion, anxiety, nervousness, abnormal dreams.
- GI: diarrhea, nausea, vomiting, constipation, abdominal pain

Serious side effects:

Vigabatrin may cause permanent vision loss at any time during treatment, as well as psychosis, depression and agitation.

Other AEDs that can increase the blood level of vigabatrin:

None anticipated

Other AEDs that can decrease the blood level of vigabatrin:

None anticipated

Other drug interactions:

None anticipated

Who should *not* take this medication?

Do not take vigabatrin if you have:
- Allergies to vigabatrin

- Absence and myoclonic seizures, as it may worsen these conditions

Note: Those with a history of psychiatric illness should use with caution.

Valproic Acid (1978)
Brand name(s):

Depakene®, Depakote®, Depakote ER®, Depakote Sprinkle®, Depakon® (injectable)

Author's opinion:

Valproic acid is an excellent first-line medication but has some side effects that limit its use. Women of childbearing age should use it with caution as it may cause birth defects and other pregnancy complications more frequently than other medications do.

Type of epilepsy it helps:

Partial and generalized; multiple seizure types

Other uses:

Bipolar disorder, migraines

Method of administration:

Valproic acid is taken via tablet, capsule, extended-release capsule, delayed-release capsule, oral suspension or injection. Extended release capsules are taken once a day, the other forms are taken 2 or more times a day. The oral forms are always better absorbed when taken with food.

Average dose:

Initial dose is 10-15 mg/kg/day (divided doses; 2-3 times/day); increased by 5-10 mg/kg/week to a final dose below 60 mg/kg/day.

How long before it produces a steady effect?

2-5 days

Blood work needed:

Blood work is recommended every 4-6 months to monitor blood cells and liver function, among others. Monitoring blood levels of medication can help to guide treatment.

Possible side effects:

- Blood: low platelets
- Brain: tremor, drowsiness, dizziness, hearing loss, insomnia, nervousness, and depression.
- GI: diarrhea, nausea, vomiting, abdominal pain, increased appetite, weight gain, potential liver and pancreas toxicity.
- Other: hair loss

Note: Hair loss and pancreatic toxicity may be reduced by supplementing with zinc and selenium. Liver toxicity may be reduced by supplementing with carnitine.

Serious side effects:

- Inflammation of the pancreas,
- Liver disease and/or liver failure (especially under age 2 years old, on multiple AED's, with congenital metabolic disorders)
- Neural tube defects such as spina bifida in the fetus
- Polycystic ovary syndrome
- Risk of suicidal thoughts or behavior

Other AEDs that can increase the blood levels of valproic acid:

Felbamate (Felbatol®)

Other AEDs that can decrease the blood levels of valproic acid:

Carbamazpine (Tegretol® and Carbatrol®), ethosuximide (Zarontin®), phenobarbital (luminal®), phenytoin (Dilantin®), primidone (Mysoline®) and topiramate (Topamax®)

Other drug interactions:

Valproic acid increases levels of:

- AEDs: carbamazepine (Tegretol®, Carbatrol®), diaz-epam (Valium®), etosuximide (Zarontin®), lamotrigine (Lamictal®), lorazepam (Ativan®), phenytoin (Dilantin®), phenobarbital (Luminal®) and primidone (Mysoline®)
- Antidepressants: amitriptyline (Elavil®) and nortriptyline (Pamelor®)
- Antivirals: zidovudine (AZT®)

Note: Valproic acid increases the risk of allergic reaction when combined with lamotrigine (Lamictal®).

Who should *not* take this medication?

Do not take valproic acid if you have:
- Allergies to this medication
- Any serious liver problems

Zonisamide (2000)
Brand name(s):

Zonegran®

Author's opinion:

Zonisamide is a first-line medication. Some side effects need to be monitored, including problems with cognition and kidney stones.

Type of epilepsy it helps:

Partial and generalized epilepsy

Method of administration:

Capsule taken once or twice daily with or without food

Average dose:

Initial dose is 100mg daily; increased after 2 weeks to 200 mg/day for a period of at least two weeks. It can be then be increased to 300 mg/day then 400 mg/day, with each dose stable for at least two weeks moving to the next level.

How long does it take to start having a steady effect?

Up to 2 weeks (approximately 10 days)

Blood work needed:

Periodic (4-6 months) blood work is recommended to check blood cells and liver function among others.

Possible side effects:

- Brain: confusion, irritability, difficulty thinking, lack of coordination
- GI: gastritis, gastric discomfort, weight loss
- Other: kidney stones, decreased sweating

Serious side effects:

- Allergic reactions

Other AEDs that can increase the blood level of zonisamide:

None anticipated

Other AEDs that can decrease the blood level of zonisamide:

Carbamazepine (Tegretol®, Carbatrol®), phenobarbital (Luminal®), phenytoin (Dilantin®), primidone (Mysoline®) and, valproic acid (Depakote®)

Other drug interactions:

None anticipated

Who should *not* take this medication?

Caution when combined with other medications that could possibly worsen metabolic acidosis. (acetazolamide or topiramate)

BENZODIAZEPINES

The benzodiazepines are best known for their ability to produce sedation, induce sleep and relieve anxiety and muscle spasms, but they also have anti-seizure effects and can be used in the short-term for epilepsy. They are not usually long term therapy because they cause drowsiness and tolerance. (The body gets used to these medications over time and needs higher and higher doses to achieve the same effects.) The only benzodiazepine that is sometimes used long-term is clobazam (Frisium®), as it may take longer to develop a tolerance to this medication.

Benzodiazepines are mainly used to abort seizures, especially when a seizure is very prolonged or several seizures have occurred in succession (seizure clusters). Administered orally or rectally, the benzodiazepines enter the system rapidly and are very effective at stopping seizures in progress. Unfortunately, all benzodiazepines cause drowsiness and may slow the rate of breathing; thus they should be used only under strict medical supervision. When these medications are suddenly discontinued, seizures are likely to recur, so they must be withdrawn gradually.

Benzodiazepines - General and Specific

General - Type of epilepsy helped:
Partial and generalized epilepsy.

General - Other uses:
Anxiety; some are also used during alcohol detoxification

General - Side effects include:
Drowsiness, fatigue, lack of coordination, increased salivation, increased urination.

More rarely there may be a loss of sexual interest, lack of motivation and memory problems. Benzodiazepines may also worsen depression.

General - Serious side effects include:
- Allergic reactions
- Breathing difficulties
- Excessive sleepiness
- Risk of suicidal thoughts or behavior

General - Common drug interactions:

The actions of the benzodiazepines may be increased by:
- Alcohol
- Barbiturates
- Monoamine oxidase inhibitors or other antidepressants.
- Narcotics
- Phenothiazines

Below is information on specific benzodiazepines (some of the most commonly used to control seizures).

General - Who should not take this medication?

Benzodiazepines should be used with caution if you have:
- Acute narrow angle glaucoma.
- Allergies to this medication
- Liver or kidney disease (significant)
- Myasthenia gravis
- Respiratory problems

Note: These medications must not be combined with alcohol, as fatal overdoses can occur.

Clobazam (2011)
Brand name(s):

Frisium®

Method of administration:

Tablet taken one to three times a day with or without food

Average dose:
- Children: is usually started at 5 mg per day and can be increased weekly by 5 mg up to 1 mg/kg
- Adults: usually started at 10 mg and can be increased after a week. Rarely more than 30 mg per day.

How long before it produces a steady effect?

One or more weeks

AEDs that can increase the blood level of clobazam:

Valproic acid (Depakote®)

AEDs that can decrease the blood level of clobazam:

Carbamazepine (Tegretol®, Carbatrol®), phenytoin (Dilantin®)

Other medications that affect clobazam:

Alcohol and an antacid cimetidine (Tagamet®) increase the level of clobazam .

Clonazepam (1975)
Brand name(s):

Klonopin®

Method of administration:

Tablet and wafers, taken one to three times a day with or without food

Average dose:

- Children: Initial dose is 0.01-0.03 mg/kg/day (in divided doses); maintenance dose is 0.1-0.2 mg/kg/day
- Adults: Initial dose is .25 mg/day; maintenance dose is 4-20 mg/day (in divided doses) Start with .25 mg, then slowly increase by increments of 0.5-1 mg every three days; dosage should not exceed 20 mg/day.

How long before it produces a steady effect?

Two or more weeks

AEDs that can increase the blood level of clonazepam:

None anticipated

AEDs that can decrease the blood level of clonazepam:

Carbamazepine (Tegretol®, Carbatrol®), phenytoin (Dilantin®)

Clorazepate
Brand name(s):

Tranxene®

Method of administration:

Tablet (one to 3 times a day)

Average dose:

- Children: Initial dose is 7.5 mg (in divided doses); dose should not exceed 60 mg/day. Not recommended for children under age 9.
- Adults: Initial dose is 7.5 mg (in divided doses); dose should not exceed 90 mg/day

How long before it produces a steady effect?

2 days to weeks

AEDs that can increase the blood level of clorazepate:

None anticipated

AEDs that can decrease the blood level of clorazepate:

None anticipated

Diazepam (1963)
Brand name(s):

Valium®

Method of administration:

Tablet, extended release tablet, liquid and injection, taken with or without food.

Average dose:

- Children: Initial dose is 1 mg to 2.5 mg, 3 - 4 times daily; increased gradually as needed
- Adults: 2 mg to 10 mg, 2 to 4 times daily

How long before it produces a steady effect?

12 to 24 hours

AEDs that can increase the blood level of diazepam:

None anticipated

AEDs that can decrease the blood level of diazepam:

None anticipated

Lorazepam
Brand name(s):

Ativan®

Method of administration:

Tablet or oral liquid, taken with or without food.

Average dose:

This medication is usually reserved for emergency purposes and the dosage varies according to weight. The doctor will customize for each patient.

How long before it produces a steady effect?

1-5 days

AEDs that can increase the blood level of lorazepam:

Valproic acid (Depakote®)

AEDs that can decrease the blood level of lorazepam:

None anticipated

CHAPTER SEVEN
SURGERY

While up to 70 percent of people with epilepsy can control their seizures through medication, some 30 percent find that medication either doesn't work or produces unacceptable side effects. In such cases, surgical removal of the area in the brain where the seizure originates may be an option.

The decision to undergo brain surgery to control your epilepsy is most certainly a major one. *Any* surgery carries with it the risk of complications and side effects, but when it involves your brain, the smallest risk can seem gargantuan. Obviously the benefits would have to be tremendous for you to even *think* about having brain surgery – and fortunately, they can be. In some cases, surgery can result in significant improvement in seizure control or even permanent freedom from seizures.

But who should consider surgery? And under what circumstances? A general rule of thumb is that surgery should be considered *only* after a patient has tried three major anticonvulsant medications without a satisfactory response. If three medications have failed to control the disorder, the odds of a fourth one working are less than five percent.

Among those who are good candidates for surgery and have a type of epilepsy that responds well to this form of treatment, quality of life may be the deciding factor. That is, if the quality of life has become unacceptable due to uncontrollable seizures, surgery may be a logical next step. Of course, just how "acceptable" a person finds his or her quality of life is a highly personal decision. For some, one uncontrollable seizure per year may be unacceptable because it's enough to prevent them from driving and, possibly, working. For others, several seizures a day might be more acceptable than undergoing brain surgery.

Whether or not surgery is right for you is a decision that only you and your doctor can make together. You will be in a much better position to make this major decision once you become familiar with the kinds of surgeries, possible benefits and risks, and the situations most likely to lead to surgical success. In this chapter, you'll learn about the surgeries that may control or even cure epilepsy, their possible complications, what makes a person a good surgical candidate, and the tests that indicate whether or not surgery might be a viable option.

There are two main kinds of surgical procedures for epilepsy: brain resection and stimulator implantation. A brain resection is the removal of a part of the brain or scar tissue or something that has invaded the brain, such as a tumor. In stimulator implantation, nothing is removed from the brain. Instead, a device is implanted in the body that delivers electrical impulses to the brain that are designed to interfere with a seizure. Let's take a closer look at these two types of surgery.

SURGICAL RESECTIONS: REMOVING A PART OF THE BRAIN

When I first suggested surgery to Mark, a 38 year-old patient of mine who had been having seizures since he was three months old, he didn't know what to think. It sounded so drastic and terrifying. He resisted the idea for an entire next year, during which his seizures got worse, sometimes occurring every hour. Then one day a life-threatening seizure propelled him into the middle of traffic on a busy street, where he just missed getting hit by a car. He called me immediately and said, "I want that surgery." He underwent a brain resection two months later, and to say that it was successful is an understatement. His seizures completely disappeared and his entire life opened up. Today, Mark has been seizure-free for 13 years and does things he never dreamed of in the past: driving, taking the train alone, working at a challenging job, going on cruises and living a completely independent life. He describes himself as "a whole new person" who has truly been "born again."

It sounds radical to the extreme: cutting away a part of your brain to keep your seizures at bay. And while any surgery to the brain certainly *is* a drastic measure, in many well-selected cases it works amazingly well. There are several different types of resections, ranging from excising a very tiny tumor to removing literally half of the brain. These procedures include lesionectomy, non-lesional resection, lobectomy, hemispherectomy, corpus callosotomy and multiple subpial transection.

Lesionectomy

Literally the cutting away of a lesion ("wound"), this surgery involves the removal of an area in the brain that has been damaged or functions abnormally. Examples of lesions include tumors, scars resulting from infections or head injuries, abnormal blood vessels and hematomas (bruises to the brain). When a lesion is causing the seizures, its removal may bring about a cure. Some 60 to 80 percent of lesionectomies result in seizure freedom or significant improvement in the seizure disorder.

Non-Lesional Resection

This surgery involves the removal of the area of the brain where the seizure originates (the seizure focus), even though there is no visible lesion. There is, however, electrical activity in that area that is clearly causing the seizures. If the seizure focus is located in the temporal lobe, there is a 70-80 percent chance of becoming seizure-free. If it is located in the other lobes, the odds of seizure freedom are around 30 to 60 percent.

Lobectomy

The brain is divided into four lobes: temporal, frontal, parietal and occipital. Partial seizures arise from one of these four lobes and cause symptoms related to the functions governed by that area (e.g. memory and hearing in the temporal lobe; movement and planning in the frontal lobe; touch in the parietal lobe; and vision in the occipital lobe). Speech is located in the frontal and temporal lobes, usually on the left side. One or part of these four lobes is removed during a lobectomy.

Three out of ten people who have temporal lobe epilepsy do not respond to standard medical treatment and may be candidates for surgery. Of those with temporal lobe epilepsy who do undergo surgery, approximately 60 to 80 percent experience seizure freedom or significant improvement in the seizure disorder. Similar results are seen in frontal, parietal or occipital lobe surgery if there is a clear lesion. Without a clear lesion, however, the rate drops to 30-60 percent.

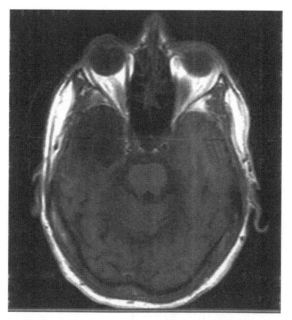

MRI showing a brain after brain surgery on the right temporal lobe

Hemispherectomy

For a hemispherectomy, one entire hemisphere (half) of the brain is removed. This surgery is performed when the seizures are so devastating that removal of a large portion of the brain is preferable to having seizures, even though the surgery will result in functional deficits.

The good news is if a hemispherectomy is performed at young age (usually before the patient is 7 years old), most of the brain function will be recovered. This is due to "brain plasticity," a phenomenon occurring in very young brains that allows functionality to shift to an intact part of the brain. For example, a young child undergoing a hemispherectomy will be paralyzed on one side immediately after the surgery, but in a few months will slowly start recovering movement as the remaining half of the brain "takes on new duties." Unfortunately, brain plasticity is not seen in adults to the same degree.

Fifty to 80 percent of those undergoing hemispherectomies experience seizure freedom or significant improvement in the seizure disorder.

Corpus Callosotomy

The two halves of the brain are connected by fibers called the corpus callosum. These fibers form the major "highway" that allows information to pass from one half of the brain to the other. During this surgery, the corpus callosum is cut, which reduces the severity of the seizures because they can no longer spread from one half of the brain to the other. The corpus callosotomy does not always eliminate seizures, as they can still originate on one side of the brain or the other. But it decreases their severity as they can no longer race across the "highway" to invade the other side.

This surgery is designed for those who cannot undergo a focal resection or even a lobectomy because there is no single seizure focus. It works very well in those with seizures producing a sudden loss of muscle tone and "drop attacks," with 50 to 70 percent of cases experiencing seizure freedom or significant improvement in the seizure disorder.

Multiple Subpial Transection (MST)

While the corpus callosotomy severs the connections between one half of the brain and the other, MST seeks to short-circuit seizures by cutting nerve fibers that link the brain's inner and outer layers. MST doesn't eliminate seizures, but does prevent them from spreading from a seizure focus in the outer layers to the deeper layers of the brain where vital functions are controlled. . The neurosurgeon does not remove any part of the brain but instead makes small cuts (transections) that do not go deep, and reach only through gray matter. This type of procedure disrupts the communication between nerve cells responsible for seizures without disrupting the communication needed for adequate function. MST is usually used to treat seizures in areas of brain that have important function.

MST is mainly performed on patients with Landau-Kleffner syndrome, a type of epilepsy seen in children that causes a loss of the ability to speak or epilepsy in functional parts of the brain such as the area that controls the leg.

IS RESECTION A VIABLE OPTION FOR YOU?

Generally, two things should be true if you are seriously considering surgical resection:

1. **All (or the majority) of the seizures should arise from the same part of the brain.**

2. **No important functions should be located in the part of the brain to be removed.**

Finding the source of the epilepsy is key. If it occurs in a definable area and can be removed without significantly damaging surrounding tissue, it is highly likely that the surgery will be successful. A good candidate for surgery is a person whose seizures originate in a part of the brain where there is no function. Then the problem area can be safely excised without causing damage or a loss of function.

But if the seizure focus is widespread, indefinable, or requires surgery that would damage functional healthy brain tissue (e.g. it is located in the part of the brain that controls movement of the legs), then the surgery may be unsuccessful or produce unacceptable side effects. A poor candidate for surgery is a person with seizures that originate in an area that governs an important function, or arise from many areas, making it impossible to remove all of them.

However, when seizures are devastating and cannot be controlled in any other way, in rare occasions, some may choose to live with a deficit (for example, paralysis on one side of the body) in exchange for control of the seizures. In this case, surgery may be performed despite the fact that the seizures arise in many areas of the brain and/ or removing these tissues would impair or eliminate function.

Functional and Non-Functional Areas of the Brain

Most people think that all areas of the brain are necessary for normal day-to-day functioning, and that surgically removing any part will cause extremely negative effects. Certainly there *are* areas of the brain that are supremely important, and if brain cells or their fibers are cut, or the area is removed, major problems will occur.

But there are other parts of the brain that can be removed safely without any notable changes or loss. In some cases, other parts of the brain can perform the same functions and "take up the slack." In other cases, there may be some minor problems, but they will not be obvious. For example, removing a part of the parietal lobe could leave a blind spot in the lower corner of your field of vision, but this most likely would not be noticeable or affect your daily activities.

Areas that we wouldn't want to upset include portions of the frontal lobes (which govern the movement of body parts), areas of the parietal lobe (which govern touch), parts of the temporal lobe (which govern memory and hearing), and areas in the occipital lobe (which govern sight).

We also take care to preserve the area that controls speech, although this area varies from person to person. For example, the ability to produce speech is always located in the frontal lobe, and the ability to understand spoken words is always located in the temporal lobe. These areas reside in the left hemisphere in those who are right-handed, but they can reside in either the right or left hemisphere in those who are left-handed. We are very careful to avoid these important areas during surgery whenever possible.

TESTS

In most cases, before recommending surgery we try to ensure that the problem is localized and has a specific source, and that removing a portion of the brain or cutting nerve fibers won't produce much (if any) collateral damage. We do this by administering various tests designed to answer the following questions:

Do the Seizures Arise From One Place?
In order to answer this question we have to perform many tests:

- **Video-EEG monitoring** - We begin with the video-EEG monitoring to determine the location of the excessive electrical activity in the brain (the seizure focus). As a general rule, the more seizures that are recorded, the more certain we are of where they begin; thus, we need to record at least 3-5 seizures. Then we compare the video portion of the test to the EEG portion to see what the patient is doing physically during the seizure, which can help us better determine where the seizure is coming from. If the seizure focus is located in just one part of the brain (rather than several), the patient might be a candidate for surgery. Additional tests that might be used include:

- **Magnetoencephalogram (MEG)** - Rather than detecting electrical fields, the MEG captures the magnetic fields of the brain. This could provide information not supplied by the regular EEG, because the MEG allows us to "see" deep into the brain. The MEG is mainly used to show the activity in the brain in between the seizures. Because it is a very expensive machine, most centers do not have one.

We can also use these imaging studies to find and "map out" the seizure focus:

- **High resolution MRI** - MRI is an essential device of imaging for epilepsy, and this sophisticated version can show very small lesions like scar tissue or tiny brain malformations that cannot be seen on a standard MRI. This improves the ability to identify the seizure focus and determine whether or not a patient is a candidate for surgical treatment.

- **Magnetic resonance spectroscopy (MRS)** – While the MRI tells us about the structure of body tissues, the MRS provides information about its biochemistry. MRS measures the levels of certain chemical compounds in the brain and helps to quantify the level of brain damage, if any, by indicating the amount of scar tissue versus the amount of total brain cells.

- **Positron emission tomography (PET scan)** - While the standard MRI works well for discovering and delineating lesions (a lesion may contribute to a seizure without actually causing it.), the PET scan can help pinpoint the seizure focus by assessing the amount of glucose (sugar) used by various areas of the brain. Every part of the brain regularly uses glucose to function. But areas that are damaged and contain fewer brain cells might use less glucose or none at all. The PET scan will highlight differently for these areas, indicating possible points of seizure origin.

Technically, the test involves the injection of a dye containing glucose that emits a low dose of radiation which is administered when the patient is not having seizures. Because the tracer contains glucose, it is consumed by the brain cells. A brain scan is then performed to see if any areas are consuming lesser amounts of the tracer, referred to as "cold" (hypometabolic) areas. Such an area may be the seizure focus.

- **Single photon emission computed tomography (SPECT scan)** - The SPECT scan measures blood flow to areas of the brain. During a seizure, the part of the brain that is more active than the rest of the brain – and takes more blood flow – is called "hyperperfusion area" and indicates the location of seizure origin. The SPECT scan is then performed between seizures, and blood flow measurements of both are compared to note the difference.

Is the Surgery Safe?

Several tests can be done to evaluate brain function and locate important parts of the brain, such as speech and memory centers. This information helps the surgeon avoid inflicting brain damage during surgery, ensuring a safer surgery with a better outcome.

- **Neuropsychological testing** - This series of oral, written and computerized tests provides information on how the brain is functioning and the cognitive strengths and weaknesses of the patient. The areas assessed include intelligence, attention, memory, speech, visual perception, motor skills and processing information. Administered by a psychologist who specializes in neuropsychological testing with special training in epilepsy, the tests can take from 3 to 8 hours.

These tests can help confirm the location of the focus. For example, if we suspect a left temporal focus and the patient has verbal memory and word finding problems (which originate in the left temporal lobe), it reassures us that our suspected focus is on target. Or, let's say we plan to remove the right temporal lobe and the patient is having a problem with verbal memory. This tells us that the left temporal lobe may also not be working properly and may predict problems after surgery. Since the left temporal lobe will be the only part left that supports memory and it is showing deficits this will be of concern.

- **Functional MRI** - A standard MRI shows the structure of the brain, while a functional MRI (fMRI) shows how the brain is functioning. It is used to locate important parts of the brain, such as the speech and movement centers, and show where these areas are in relation to the seizure focus. During the fMRI, the patient is asked to perform some simple tasks and answer some questions. The functional MRI will map which parts of the brain "light up" while certain tasks are completed, which helps determine which parts of the brain house which functions.

- **Wada test (Amytal test)** - This test, first described by an epilepsy specialist named Dr. Jung Wada, helps determine which half of the brain handles which functions. For the test, a catheter is inserted in the groin area and guided upward into one of the two carotid arteries, the major blood vessels in the neck that bring blood to the brain. A barbiturate (usually Amytal) is then injected into the carotid artery and carried to one half of the brain, putting just that half to sleep. This allows the doctor to assess how the other half of the brain functions all by itself.

At this point, the patient's speech and memory are assessed. If the speech area is located in the "sleeping" half of the brain, the patient will not be able to respond verbally.

Memory is assessed by showing objects to the patient while under the influence of the barbiturate, then asking him or her to recall and recognize the objects once the brain "wakes up." This information is very important in the planning of the surgery. If we plan to remove part of the left half of the brain, for example, we want to make sure that the right side has healthy memory/speech functions so the patient will still be able to speak and form memories after the surgery.

Additional "invasive" testing is only used when the exact seizure focus is not being detected or when doctors need to make sure that important functions would not be damaged with surgery.

- **Subdural electrodes** – placing subdural electrodes on the surface of the brain (a grid of electrodes is "implanted" through a surgical procedure) allow to:

    o Localize seizure focus with more precision since the electrodes are in direct contact with the brain
    o Map important functions of the brain (i.e. speech and movements) by giving a specific and very small part of the brain an electrical charge to see the effects

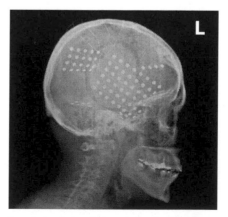

Skull x-ray showing subdural electrode placed to map the seizure focus and functional parts of the brain

- **Depth electrodes** – are electrodes placed within the brain to localize seizure focus in a very precise manner

Surgery Complications and Failure

Like every other surgery, those performed to control or eliminate epileptic seizures can produce complications, although they are rare. There may be problems related to anesthesia, which can result in death. There is always a possibility of accidentally nicking an artery or a vein which, in extreme cases, could result in a stroke. And there is a risk of infection, particularly when electrodes are used on or in the brain. The longer the electrodes are used, the greater the chances of infection.

There is also a chance that the surgery will not improve or eliminate the seizures. This can occur for several reasons: the seizure focus was not correctly identified or removed; removal of the entire seizure focus was impossible because it was located in an area that governed important function; there was a second epileptic focus that was not previously identified and therefore not removed; or the surgeon did not remove all of the targeted brain tissue. However, as long as the patient is a good candidate for surgery, proper testing has been completed and standard surgical techniques are employed, the vast majority of surgeries to control epilepsy are successful.

Post-Surgery Protocol

Generally, after brain surgery it is recommended that the patient rest at home for a month and engage in minimal activity. A return to work and normal activities is usually possible in three months, provided there are no complications.

STIMULATOR IMPLANTATION

By now you may be wondering if there is some way to control your seizures *other* than brain surgery! What happens if you're not candidate for brain surgery, no surgery exists that is right for your condition, or you just plain don't want to have your brain operated on? The answer may be *vagus nerve stimulation* (VNS), a pacemaker-like device inserted in the body that generates pulses of electricity that interfere with seizures. VNS was approved by the FDA in 1997 as a treatment for partial-onset seizures in those 12 and older whose seizures haven't responded to medication.

How Does the VNS Work?

The VNS emits pulses of electricity that stimulate the vagus nerve, a major nerve that conducts impulses between the brain and various organs/structures including the larynx, heart, lungs and gastrointestinal tract. Scientists have known since the 1930's that stimulating the vagus nerve causes EEG changes, but using this technique to reduce seizures did not occur until 1988. Since that time, studies have shown that most patients using VNS experience a reduction in seizures of more than 50 percent after 18 months of treatment.

The battery-operated vagus nerve stimulator, a device that resembles a silver dollar in size and shape, is implanted through the skin of the upper chest. Wires are threaded from the implant through the neck and wrapped around the vagus nerve, a cranial nerve that passes from the abdomen through the chest and neck carrying electrical impulses to the brain. The surgery can be done on an outpatient basis and takes approximately an hour.

The VNS is programmed to deliver a set amount of electrical stimulation to the vagus nerve at certain intervals around the clock. A common pattern is 30 seconds of stimulation every 5 minutes. The doctor will often change the amount and frequency of stimulation, slowly raising the settings, which means the patient will need to see the doctor often for VNS adjustments.

A special magnet can also be used to exert some control over the VNS. This magnet, which is worn like a wristwatch, delivers extra electrical stimulation when passed over the area where the VNS is implanted. The additional stimulation may be enough to abort a seizure that has just started or ward off one that's about to start. The magnet can also have the opposite effect: When steadily holding it over the device, it will turn off the stimulation for awhile. This could be helpful if the patient's throat has become irritated from the stimulation and is having difficulty eating or is about to make a speech. (See "Adverse Effects" below.)

Adverse Effects

Since the vagus nerve controls the larynx ("voice box"), the VNS can irritate this organ and cause coughing, vocal changes, hoarseness and pharyngitis. Fortunately, these symptoms can usually be relieved by decreasing the intensity of the VNS impulses. Sleep apnea, although rare, may also occur.

Warning!

- If you have a VNS device implanted, do not get an MRI that involves the use of a body coil, as the heat it generates can cause severe damage to nerves and other tissues. (MRIs that use head coils are acceptable.) If an MRI is needed, consult your neurologist.
- Do not use deep-heat treatments for pain or wound healing, as they too can cause nerve and tissue damage.

Who Might Benefit from VNS?

VNS has been approved for treatment of partial-onset epilepsy, but it has also been used successfully for treatment of generalized epilepsy, in particular Lennox-Gastaut syndrome, as well as depression. Potentially, it could work for any type of epilepsy, but it may be particularly attractive to those who cannot or do not want to undergo brain surgery. Studies are currently underway testing the effects of VNS on anxiety disorders, migraines, Alzheimer's disease, tinnitus and fibromyalgia.

Of those who use VNS, one-third improve significantly, one-third improve somewhat, and one third do not improve at all. Becoming completely seizure-free is very rare. It's interesting to note, however, that even in those whose seizures do not improve, there can be an increase in well-being since VNS may exert a positive effect on the mood.

NEUROSTIMULATION - EXPERIMENTAL TREATMENTS FOR EPILEPSY

Ongoing epilepsy medical research has produced exciting new possibilities. One of these is neurostimulation, or electrical therapy to the brain, currently a common treatment for Parkinson's Disease and Essential Tremor.

A company called Medtronic® has completed clinical trials using deep brain stimulation for patients with treatment-resistant partial epilepsy. Throughout the duration of the study, electrodes implanted on both sides of the brain delivered electrical impulses that were shown to produce modest improvements in seizure control.

Another company, Neuropace, Inc. has completed clinical trials with its Responsive Neurostimulator® device. The device was tested on patients suffering from treatment-resistant partial epilepsy who had one or two well-defined seizure-generating areas in the brain. Electrodes were placed over these areas and connected to a small computer implanted in the skull. The computer was programmed to recognize seizure activity and respond by delivering electrical impulses. In a pivotal trial, seizure frequency was reduced by 37.9% in those using the device, compared to 17.3% receiving a sham therapy. Because these devices are currently being reviewed by the Food and Drug Administration, they are not yet available for clinical use. However these and other experimental therapies are being tested on epilepsy patients in clinical trials.

Because these devices are only available to you if you participate in such a study, at some point you may consider enrolling. I must urge you, however, to think carefully before signing on. Because the treatment is experimental, all potential risks have not yet been identified. (However, you will be closely observed by the medical team, who will remove you from the study if any side effects appear harmful.) On the positive side, you will have early access to a new treatment and may find that it offers greater relief from your symptoms. And you might help other epilepsy patients by "blazing a trail" that leads to more effective seizure control. Clearly, it is a decision that requires much thought and research before you can come up with the "right" answer for you.

CHAPTER EIGHT
DIET THERAPY

Wouldn't be great if all you had to do was eat plenty of vegetables and fish oil, or avoid chocolate and alcohol, and your seizures would just melt into the background? I'm often asked if there are any foods that are "good" or "bad" for seizures. Unfortunately, there aren't any *specific* foods that can help prevent seizures, although certain diets may be helpful. There are, however, a few foods and food additives that can *contribute* to seizures and should be approached with caution. They include:

- *Caffeine* – Because it is a stimulant, caffeine may lower the seizure threshold by contributing to the release of excitatory neurochemicals that increase the rate of nerve firing. And it can be double-trouble for those with epilepsy because caffeine can disrupt sleep, leading to insomnia, which increases the risk for seizures.

- *Energy drinks* – These drinks, which are used to increase alertness and energy levels, typically contain large amounts of caffeine, sugar, taurine, and legal herbal stimulants such as guarana seed extract and ginseng. Because of their highly stimulating effects, they have been linked to seizures in some people. Since energy drinks have no health benefits and may trigger seizures, they should be avoided completely.

- *Grapefruit and grapefruit juice* – Grapefruit slows the breakdown of the AED carbamazepine (Tegretol®), causing levels of this medication to build up in the bloodstream. This can lead to side effects such as slurred speech, difficulty balancing, nausea/vomiting, seizures, and loss of consciousness.

- *Gluten* – This special type of protein, found in wheat, barley and rye, can cause seizures in people who have gluten sensitivities. Celiac disease, the most common type of gluten intolerance, is an abnormal immune reaction to partially-digested gluten fragments. This reaction causes intestinal damage, digestive problems and, sometimes, seizures. In these cases, adopting a gluten-free diet may be enough to keep seizures at bay.

- *High sugar foods* – People with epilepsy who also have diabetes should avoid eating high sugar foods, as blood sugar that rises too high or plummets too low can trigger seizures. .

- *Certain other foods* – Foods that have been suggested (but not proven) to be seizure triggers include wheat, soy, dairy and MSG. Interestingly, all of these products contain high amounts of glutamine, a substance with an excitatory effect on the brain that could bring on seizures.

ANTI-SEIZURE DIETS

While no specific food has been proven to lessen or prevent epileptic seizures, the ketogenic diet, the modified Atkins diet and the low glycemic index diet may be useful in treating epilepsy. These diets all produce a similar result: a metabolic state known as *ketosis*. In its normal state, the body burns carbohydrates (glucose and glycogen) for fuel. But during ketosis, the fuel source becomes the body's fat stores. Ketones are little carbon fragments created from the breakdown of fat that the body uses as an energy source. *Ketosis* occurs when ketones build up to a certain level in the blood.

In order to put the body into ketosis, the carbohydrate supply must be severely limited, since the body will always opt to burn carbohydrates if they're available. It's only when both dietary carbohydrate (sugars and starches) and carbohydrate stored in the body (glycogen) are depleted or unavailable that the body shifts gears and starts burning fat for energy and producing ketones. Amazingly, in some patients ketones have a protective effect against seizures! And in some, this effect may continue even after the diet has been discontinued.

Ketogenic Diet

While some diets produce ketosis as a "side effect," the purpose of the ketogenic diet is to cultivate and maintain this metabolic state. The diet was first used to treat epilepsy in the 1920s, but it wasn't until the 1990's that the ketogenic diet became widely known, thanks to Hollywood producer Jim Abrahams. His toddler son Charlie suffered multiple daily epileptic seizures that did not respond to medications. The child even underwent brain surgery, to no avail. Yet Charlie's epilepsy was stopped through the use of the ketogenic diet, which prompted Abrahams to make a movie about the diet called "First, Do No Harm" that starred Meryl Streep. He also created The Charlie Foundation, a nonprofit organization that raises awareness about the ketogenic diet and sponsors new research on this topic.

In a nutshell, the ketogenic diet is very high in fat, provides sufficient protein to prevent protein-energy malnutrition, and severely restricts carbohydrate. Due to the limited types of foods allowed on this diet, almost all patients are advised to use vitamin and mineral supplements. (Each patient's registered dietitian will determine which supplements are needed.) To ensure ketosis at all times, the amount of fat consumed must be 3 to 4 times greater than the combination of carbohydrate and protein consumed, gram for gram. All foods and most drinks must be weighed on a gram scale to ensure accuracy and protein intake must also be monitored very closely.

The Ketogenic Ratio

The ketogenic ratio is a comparison of the amount of fat to the amount of protein/carbohydrate in the diet. The ratio is determined by weight (in grams), *not* calories, with a typical ketogenic diet containing 3 grams fat per 1 gram of protein and/or carbohydrate (3:1). The higher the ratio, the more ketone bodies will be produced, and the more "ketogenic" the diet. Typical ketogenic diets have ratios that range from 2:1 to 5:1, although anything greater than 4.1 is very difficult to achieve (except through tube feeding) because food choices become so restricted.

A enteral (feeding tube) formula called Ketocal, available in liquid and powdered form, comes in a 4:1 ratio. The powdered form, which is used for both oral and tube feeding, must be weighed on a gram scale. It can also be used as a baking agent to make foods like pancakes, muffins, cake, and smoothies.

Non-food items must also be taken into account on the ketogenic diet. Believe it or not, medications, shampoos, lotions, sunscreens and several other household products contain carbohydrates that can be absorbed through the skin or digestive tract! Medications must be compounded into a carbohydrate-free form and only certain kinds of household items should be used. (A full list of approved household items can be found at www.charliefoundation.org.)

Getting started

If you're thinking about trying the ketogenic diet, have an initial consultation with an epileptologist that includes a screening to determine the state of your health. If all is well, the next step is a nutritional consultation with a registered dietitian with special expertise in these diets, who will explain the nuts and bolts of the diet, including food ratios, calorie requirements, and fluid intake. Pre-diet lab work must be completed to ensure that you don't have elevated cholesterol or triglyceride levels, as the diet can exacerbate these conditions. These blood tests will check if you have some of rare metabolic conditions in which this type of diet would be contraindicated. In addition, these labs are compared to the same lab values while you are on the diet. A brief hospital admission may be beneficial upon initiation of the diet in order to ensure appropriate glucose levels, stable blood work and allow time for your family/caregivers to receive further education and get more comfortable with the diet.

The method of diet initiation varies among centers. Some may ask you to fast for a day to promote ketosis, while others gradually increase the ratio of fat to carbohydrate and protein over a period of 2-4 days, with no fasting required. Recent research suggested that there is no benefit to withholding food completely, especially from children.

The ketogenic diet is usually followed until the patient becomes seizure-free, and is then continued for an additional year or longer. In most cases, an attempt to wean the patient off the diet is made after 1.5 to 2 years. The post-weaning results will vary according to the individual: some continue the success they had while on the diet, others experience a small setback in improvements, while still others see a reversal in improvements. Follow-up care includes regular visits and phone calls to the dietitian, the daily measurement of ketones in urine, and visits to the epileptologist to check lab values and growth parameters.

How effective is the diet?

Though the figures vary, studies show that the ketogenic diet is effective in approximately two thirds of the patients that try it, despite their age, although the degree of success varies from person to person. In one person, the seizures may stop completely, another may experience a 50 percent seizure reduction, while a third experiences only a 25 percent reduction. If there are no immediately apparent benefits, it is standard procedure to follow the diet for at least 8 to 12 weeks before concluding that it's ineffective. But remember that even if the diet is unsuccessful in the sense that it does not eliminate seizures, it may help enough to make it possible to reduce the dosage of AEDs, lessening the chances of medication side effects.

Who is a good candidate for this diet?

The ketogenic diet is most often used in children who are not responding to medications (two to three medications have failed), or when patients/parents would rather not use medications. In childhood epilepsy syndromes such as Dravet Syndrome, the diet has proven to be very effective and may be considered more of a first-line treatment. And even though the ketogenic diet is mainly used in children, adults may also benefit from it.

Who is *not* a good candidate for this diet?

The ketogenic diet should be avoided by those who have pyruvate carboxylase deficiency, porphyria, or diseases involving fat metabolism. Also, anyone who doesn't have the time, dedication or discipline to follow the diet (or, for children, those who don't have highly motivated and disciplined parents) should find other, non-dietary ways to control epilepsy. Diet therapy for epilepsy must be strictly followed and taken as seriously as medication. The right proportion of fat vs. protein/carbohydrate must be provided at all times with absolutely no exceptions. Slipping in even a small carbohydrate-based treat or making a mistake in weighing foods could be enough to disrupt the entire process and bring on a seizure.

Foods That Contain Carbohydrate

Since consuming even a little bit of a carbohydrate can bring a sudden halt to ketosis and its seizure-preventing effects, it's worthwhile to take a look a closer look at what's included in this food group.

- **Starchy foods** – Bread, rolls, bagels, cereal, rice, pasta, pretzels, potato chips, crackers, waffles, pancakes, potatoes, corn, peas and beans.

- **Fruit/fruit juice** – Any kind of fresh, frozen or canned fruit or fruit juice.

- Vegetables – Any kind of fresh, frozen, or canned vegetable or vegetable juice.

- **Milk/yogurt/ice cream** – All kinds of milk, yogurt, cheese, and ice cream, including full fat, 2%, 1% and nonfat.

- **Sweets/simple sugars** – Sugar, honey, jelly, jam, syrup, BBQ sauce, ketchup, sweet pickles, sweet relish, candy, cookies, cakes, pie, brownies, chewing gum that contains sugar, sugared soft drinks.

Check out http://www.lowcarb.com for some great low carbohydrate options including low carb candies, breads and sauces. Remember all of these foods would need to be eaten with a significant amount of fat.

Side effects of the ketogenic diet

Although the ketogenic diet can be very helpful for preventing seizures, it has some potential side effects in adults and children, Including high cholesterol/triglycerides, kidney stones (usually secondary to dehydration) and acidosis (excess amounts of acid in the body fluids). In adults, menstrual irregularities, pancreatitis, bone fractures and eye problems may also occur.

Many people are concerned about the large proportion of fat in the ketogenic diet, wondering if it will contribute to weight gain and elevated cholesterol/triglyceride levels. While either can occur, especially when the diet is followed for long periods of time, results will vary according to the individual. To monitor for side effects, it's important that you see your doctor every 1-3 months for blood tests measuring cholesterol, triglycerides, liver function, electrolytes, and pancreatic enzymes. Growth in children who are following the ketogenic diet should also be assessed regularly.

Modified Atkins Diet

Although the Atkins diet for weight loss has been around since the 1970's, the modified Atkins diet, which is used specifically to control epileptic seizures, didn't appear in the scientific literature until 2003. It came about when some families using the ketogenic diet for long periods of time stopped weighing and measuring their food and noticed that ketones and seizure control remained high.

As the name suggests, modified Atkins is a version of the traditional Atkins diet, a well-known weight loss program based on higher amounts of fat and protein in the diet and lower amounts of carbohydrates. This combination produces ketosis, which promotes fat burning. The modified Atkins diet encourages fat intake more strongly than the traditional Atkins diet, and restricts carbohydrates more severely (10 g per day in children and 15 g per day in adults). In contrast, patients on a traditional Atkins diet go through phases when they may be allowed more than 20 grams of carbohydrate per day. The combination of more fat and less carbohydrate is the most likely reason that those on the modified Atkins diet produce ketones (or should be producing them), while those on the traditional Atkins diet may not.

Compared to the ketogenic diet, the modified Atkins diet is easier to follow and much more palatable, making it popular with the adult population. There are no limits regarding the intake of calories, protein or fluid, and foods are not weighed or measured, so meals can be eaten in restaurants and at other people's homes. Some carbohydrate can be consumed, although it must be monitored carefully. Finally, fasting and/or hospitalization are not required to initiate the diet. It does, however, require vitamin and mineral supplementation as well as initial and follow-up lab work and growth measurements (in children).

While not many studies have been done on the effects of the modified Atkins diet on seizures, the few that have been completed show similar results to the ketogenic diet, even though the ketogenic ratio on modified Atkins is low (typically around1:1).

Low Glycemic Index Diet

Like the previous two, the goal of the low glycemic index diet is ketosis when it's used to prevent epileptic seizures. However, this diet focuses on the *type* of carbohydrates eaten, as opposed to the amount. It does this by utilizing the glycemic index.

Originally created as a tool to help diabetics control their blood sugar levels, the glycemic index (GI) measures the increase in blood sugar produced by 50 gram portions of various types of carbohydrate, compared to the same amount of a control (pure glucose or white bread). After each food is tested, it is given a rating on a100-point index, with 100 assigned to pure glucose. High glycemic foods are those rated 70 or above; moderate glycemic foods are those rated between 56 and 69, and low glycemic foods are rated 55 or below.

When using this diet for prevention of epileptic seizures, only foods that have a low GI (less than 50) are allowed. Total carbohydrates are gradually decreased to about 10 percent of the daily calories (40-50 grams), then decreased further if seizures still occur. The carbohydrates are spread evenly throughout the day and eaten along with protein and fat to slow the release of glucose into the blood. This diet has less fat than the ketogenic diet (60-70 percent of daily calories vs. 90 percent), and more protein (20-30 percent of daily calories.)

The upshot is that the low glycemic index diet is easier to follow than the ketogenic diet because it allows more carbohydrates and protein and requires less fat. This makes the diet less restrictive, although reaching ketosis may be more difficult.

To date, there are not many studies testing the effects of the low glycemic index diet on seizures. However, one of the few studies conducted found that 10 out of 20 patients with intractable epilepsy who followed the low-glycemic index diet reduced their seizure frequency by more than 29 percent.[1] It should be noted, however, that some patients may need to increase their seizure medication while on this diet.

COMPARING THE ANTI-SEIZURE DIETS

While all three diets are designed to prevent seizures by promoting ketosis, there are differences between them in the principles and practical applications (actual food eaten), as illustrated by the following charts:

DIETARY PRINCIPLES	KETOGENIC	MODIFIED ATKINS	LOW GLYCEMIC INDEX
Low carbohydrate & high fat	Yes	Yes	Yes
Calorie restriction	Yes	No	No
Protein restriction	Yes	No	No
Food must be weighed	Yes	No	No
Based on ketogenic ratio	Yes	No	No
Hospital admission	Yes (most epilepsy centers)	No	No
Fasting required	varies among epilepsy centers	No	No

[1] Pfeifer HH, Thiele EA. Low-glycemic-index treatment: A liberalized ketogenic diet for treatment of intractable epilepsy. *Neurology* 2005;65(11):1810-12.

SAMPLE MENUS

	KETOGENIC	*MODIFIED ATKINS*	*LOW GLYCEMIC INDEX*
Breakfast	20 grams of egg 18 grams cheese 10 grams cooked bacon 6 grams butter 16 grams olive oil	Scrambled eggs made with cheese, bacon, hot tea, and water.	Broccoli and cheese omelet with 1/2 slice light whole wheat toast.
Lunch	27 grams beef bologna 5 grams mayonnaise	Chicken salad lettuce wrap (made with chicken, celery, and mayonnaise wrapped in a large leaf of lettuce)	Sliced turkey and cheese roll ups with 4 ounces of plain yogurt.
Snack	75 grams avocado 1.5 grams agave nectar	1/2 cup air popped popcorn with melted butter	Red pepper slices and 2 tablespoons hummus.
Dinner	24 grams chicken breast 15 grams cooked cauliflower 30 grams butter	Hamburger or cheeseburger with no bun, half cup broccoli, water	Pork chop with mushrooms and onions, with water or a diet beverage.
Dessert/Snack	Ketocal cranberry apple cobbler 36 grams raw apple without skin 9 grams cranberries 17 grams butter 8 grams Ketocal 4:1	Sugar free jell-o topped with heavy whipping cream	½ cup cherries

FOOD LISTS

It could take an entire chapter to list all of the foods considered permissible on each of these diets, plus all of the foods that should be limited or even eliminated. To save space, I have compiled abbreviated lists of foods that have no carbohydrate or just a trace (referred to as 100% safe foods), those with minimal carbs (questionable foods or foods you should eat with caution) and those with higher amounts of carbs (foods that may be eaten very sparingly.) Foods that are considered particularly healthy are marked with a *. I highly recommend eating these as often as possible, while keeping within your carbohydrate limits and maintaining ketosis.

100% Safe Foods (No Carbs/Trace Carbs)

Very few foods are completely "keto-friendly" (meaning they do not interfere with ketosis) without the addition of fat. For example, on the ketogenic diet, even foods with zero carbohydrate or just a tiny amount must be eaten with the correct proportion of fat. And many of these foods are very high in protein, which must be also be accounted for in the ketogenic diet. So the idea of "100% safe foods" actually means they are fine for the modified Atkins or low glycemic index diets, but they work for the ketogenic diet *only* if they are consumed with the proper proportion of additional fat and protein. Very important reminder: sugar free DOES NOT equal carbohydrate free. Examples include:

- bacon
- beef
- butter
- chicken*
- crab
- duck
- eggs
- filet mignon
- halibut*
- ham

- hamburger
- heavy cream
- lamb
- lobster
- mustard
- Nutrasweet/Equal.
- oils (olive oil*, flaxseed oil*, etc.)
- pork
- prime rib
- salmon*
- salt, pepper
- shrimp
- steak
- tea, coffee
- trout*
- tuna*

Questionable Foods (Minimal Carbs)

"Questionable" foods are those that contain some carbohydrate, but not a lot. Even though their carbohydrate content is minimal, it must be accounted for when planning a meal or snack. Label reading is a *must* as the carbohydrate content can vary widely even among the same kind of food. For example, some hot dogs contain just 1 gram of carbohydrate while others contain up to 7 grams. The following foods are among the "questionable" ones, with a carbohydrate content that must be carefully checked before eating:

- abalone
- artichokes*
- asparagus*
- bok choy*
- broccoli*
- Brussels sprouts*
- Buffalo wings
- cabbage*

- cauliflower*
- celery*
- cheese
- cucumbers*
- flaxseed*
- green beans*
- hot dogs
- kale*
- lettuce
- liverwurst
- mushrooms*
- mustard greens*
- nuts
- olives*
- onions*
- oysters
- pastrami
- peppers* (red, green, jalapeno, habanero)
- pickles
- protein powder
- ribs (watch out for the sauce!)
- salad dressing (some)
- salami
- sausage
- soy sauce
- spinach*

Higher Carb Foods (Very Limited Quantities!)

There are a few foods with a higher carbohydrate content that may be eaten in VERY limited quantities on all three diets. They include:

- all fruits*
- milk*
- all starchy products

DON'T DO IT ALONE

These three diets, especially the ketogenic diet, are *not* do-it-yourself treatments to be tried at home on your own. Diet therapy for epilepsy is a team effort that includes a registered dietitian with special expertise and knowledge in anti-seizure diets, a doctor who specializes in epilepsy, and the people who will help the patient with the day-to-day realities of living with any of these diets. This includes family members and friends, and in the case of children, teachers, babysitters, and anyone else who may be caring for them. The diet must be specifically tailored to the patient's needs, with kinds and amounts of food strictly regulated, and effects carefully monitored.

Despite the many changes that this diet requires, the results can be worth the effort.

Following the ketogenic diet, in particular, may produce long-lasting benefits, even after the diet is discontinued. Charlie Abrahams, who once had up to 100 seizures a day, has remained seizure-free since he completed the ketogenic diet in 1997. It may not work for everyone, but for some people it's nothing short of a miracle.

CHAPTER NINE
SUPPORTIVE AND COMPLEMENTARY TREATMENTS

Three year-old Nina suffered from frequent seizures that caused numerous falls and injuries. By the time her mother brought her to see me, another neurologist had been treating her seizures for years with various seizure medications. Unfortunately, they were still poorly controlled and she was in and out of emergency rooms constantly. When Nina's grandmother visited from their home country in Central America, she was appalled to learn that the child was still having seizures. She pressured her daughter to stop all of Nina's seizure medications and begin their local traditional therapy that would include prayer, herbs and different potions. Apparently Nina's uncle also had epilepsy during childhood and was treated with traditional medicine, and he no longer had seizures. Nina's mother was unsure about what to do. "I want to do what's right for my daughter," she told me. "But just giving her medicine doesn't seem to be enough."

Nina's mother was right when she said that traditional medication has limitations that can be terribly frustrating. She was also highly responsible in checking in with me before she made any changes in her daughter's treatment. At this point, our medications, surgical treatments and some specific diets are the only scientifically proven modes of treatment for epilepsy. Other treatment approaches may be useful, but we need to be clear that they remain understudied and unconfirmed.

On the other hand, while standard medical treatment certainly does help the vast majority of patients with epilepsy, no one treatment can address all the concerns associated with the disorder, including such things as memory problems, mood issues, family or social issues and the stress of dealing with a chronic condition. There are several supportive psychologically-based therapies and alternative approaches that may help alleviate specific problems that medication does not target. In this chapter, we'll review some supportive treatments and complementary/alternative medicine approaches, then take a quick look at a few experimental treatments that may soon be approved for use.

Caution: *None of these complementary treatments are meant to replace your medical treatment. Always consult your epileptologist or neurologist before beginning or ceasing any medication or treatment for your epilepsy.*

SUPPORTIVE TREATMENTS FOR EPILEPSY

Because even the best anti-seizure medicine is designed to treat seizures and nothing else, supportive treatments that improve day-to-day quality of life and psychological and mental function can be helpful and, in some cases, necessary. Several are available, the most common being psychotherapy, support groups and cognitive remediation therapy.

Psychotherapy

If epilepsy prevents you from driving, working or otherwise participating fully in life, you may experience a great sense of loss. You may find yourself feeling different or "less than" others, becoming isolated, or suffering emotionally in other ways. The loss of control that characterizes seizures can also lead to feelings of vulnerability of anxiety. Psychotherapy, especially when guided by a clinician who works regularly with epilepsy patients, can help you understand your feelings and work towards changing the ones that need to be changed in a positive direction. Therapy also offers education about epilepsy and associated depression, anxiety and other emotional issues and has many tools that the therapist can teach you for dealing effectively with these problems. Some of these tools can include relaxation techniques, assertiveness training, and learning to monitor your thoughts and feelings regularly.

Although Sarah had been diagnosed with epilepsy several years ago, only recently did she begin to experience extreme anxiety. Suddenly, she could not stop worrying about having another seizure and she couldn't tolerate being alone. Sarah's psychologist helped her realize that her anxiety stemmed from many sources, some of which had nothing to do with epilepsy. For example, she had just relocated to a new part of the country, which was stressful enough, and she was also looking hard to find a job. The psychologist taught Sarah a series of relaxation techniques that she practiced daily. Sarah also kept a journal, noting the situations and thoughts that made her start to feel nervous. Then the psychologist helped her analyze these thoughts to determine which were realistic and which were not, and helped her replace the unrealistic thoughts with those that were more rational. Once Sarah started listening to and analyzing her own thoughts, her anxiety levels decreased dramatically.

Art Therapy

Based on psychoanalytic theory, art therapy uses the techniques of drawing, painting and other forms of art to bring forth thoughts and feelings that may be buried and causing emotional stress. This could be an ideal way of receiving therapy for those who are not the "talking-type," or those who are visual and have artistic leanings.

Cognitive Remediation Therapy

People with epilepsy often complain of difficulties with memory, concentration and word finding, all of which can be related to the disorder itself, medication side effects, or associated mood problems. Cognitive remediation therapy can help you learn new strategies to improve your memory and other mental functions. Your areas of cognitive strength can be used to compensate for your areas of weakness. For example, if you have a good visual memory but have difficulty remembering verbal information (e.g. you can remember faces or colors but not names), you may learn to associate a person's name with a visual characteristic, as in "Bill wears blue a lot."

Support Groups

Support groups can offer you and your loved ones the chance to interact with people in similar situations. One of the most important benefits of a support group is the discovery that you are not alone. Other people have experienced the same things and many have regained their health and happiness – seeing this can help you keep your hopes and motivation up. Support groups can also provide a lot of useful information about epilepsy, resources, and community events.

Fran really likes her doctor, thinks that his explanations about epilepsy are clear and easy to understand, and that he offers excellent care. But her support group has given her something else: human contact with people who understand her "from the inside." When Fran is with the group, she doesn't have to explain how seizures mess up her day, or how hard it is to take all of those medications. Everybody already understands, and they offer the best practical advice there is. The group also works together as a team to do important things such as epilepsy research fundraising and epilepsy walks (once a year all the way to Washington, DC). But most of all, they offer each other friendship and support.

Psychotherapy, cognitive remediation therapy and support groups are just three of the supportive treatments available for people with epilepsy; there are others. Ask your doctor for referrals to such services in your area.

COMPLEMENTARY AND ALTERNATIVE MEDICINE IN EPILEPSY

Although traditional Western medicine has made great strides in controlling seizures, it has yet to produce the "silver bullet" that will eliminate all of them instantly and without side effects. It is also sadly lacking when it comes to delivering psychological, occupational and other forms of support. For these and other reasons, between 24 and 44 percent of those who have epilepsy turn to complementary and alternative medicine (CAM). These treatments include herbal and botanical medicine, acupuncture, magnets, chiropraxis and yoga, just to name a few.

My patients often ask me if such treatments work, and I always reply that CAM can be a very helpful adjunct to standard medicine. However – and this is an important point –

both doctor and patient *must* work together to make sure the selected CAM therapies do *not* interfere with standard treatment or produce dangerous effects.

Herbs

Herbs are the most commonly used form of CAM for epilepsy. They may also be the most ancient, having been used for centuries to treat epilepsy in Asia and other areas with established systems of Eastern medicine. Herbs that have been used to control seizures include valerian, piper nigrum, kava and withania among many others.

Many patients praise their herbal treatments, but there has been little scientific research concerning these agents. This means we really don't know if they work or not – or why they seem to work for some people but aren't helpful to others. Then there's the issue of standardization. Since herbs are not subjected to the same governmental regulations as standard medicines regarding manufacturing, purity and content, we can't say whether an herb processed by one company is just as safe or effective as the same herb processed by another company. Another risk is that some herbal supplements may contain ingredients to which you are allergic and since all the ingredients may not be listed, you would not know this.

Although there are a lot of unknowns concerning herbs, this much we can say with certainty: Many people feel their herbal treatments have helped, and many are determined to use them. Because a large number of physicians scoff at herbs, a frighteningly large number of patients don't disclose their use. This is dangerous because some herbal treatments can actually *cause* seizures, either by lowering the seizure threshold or lowering blood levels of anti-epileptic medications. So, bottom line, you need to speak to your doctor about <u>all</u> the substances you are ingesting. You may be the first person to educate your doctor about how many patients partake in herbal treatments; who knows, you may not just end up improving your own care as well as helping other fellow patients who come after you to see this same doctor.

Remember: *It is vital that doctor and patient work together when it comes to the use of herbs. Talk to your doctor before taking any herbs to make sure that, at the very least, they will not be harmful.*

Margie is a 52 year-old woman with partial seizures that have been well-controlled for many years with carbamazepine. But recently she experienced a sudden worsening in her seizures. Several months earlier Margie had begun feeling listless, lost her appetite, suffered from insomnia, and didn't even feel like knitting, which had always been her favorite hobby. She plugged her symptoms into an internet medical website and decided she was suffering from depression. When her primary care doctor recommended an antidepressant, Margie resisted because she didn't want to have to take another medication. Then she read that the herb St. John's wort had been shown to be helpful for depression. Margie ordered it online and started taking it; after several weeks, she felt less depressed. Unfortunately, she began having breakthrough seizures, and eventually ended up in the emergency room due to a seizure-related car accident. Tests showed that Margie's blood levels of carbamazepine were undetectable, resulting in the suspension of her driver's license. She found out later that St. John's wort reduces carbamazepine levels in the blood, making the medication less effective.

Warning!

Just because herbs are considered "natural" doesn't mean they can't be harmful under certain conditions, including epilepsy. Ask your doctor before taking any herbs, especially the following:

Herbs that may cause or precipitate seizures:
American hellebore
Bearberry (arcostaphyllus uva-ursi)
Borage (Borago ifficinalis)
Ephedra (ephedra)
Essential oils
Evening primrose (oenothera biennis)
Gingko (gingko)
Ginseng (Panax quinquefolius)
Hyssop (Hyssopus officinalis)
Ma Huang (herba ephedra)
Mistletoe (viscum album)
Monkshood (aconilum)
Primrose (Oenothera biennis)
Skullcap (scutellaria galericulata)
Yew (taxus bacatta)
Yohimbe (pausinystalta yohimbe)

Herbs may change the blood levels of certain AEDs:
Aloe Vera (Aloe Barbadenis)
American hellebore
Chamomile (matricaria recutita)
Echinacea (Echinacea purpurea)
Garlic (allium sativum)
Ginkgo biloba
Gotu Kola (Centella asiatica)
Kava (piper methysticum)
Licorice (Glycyrrhiza glabra)
Milk thistle (silybum marianum)
Mistletoe (viscum album)

Mugwort (Artemisia vulgaris)
Passion flower (passiflora incarnata)
Pipsissewa (chimaphila umbellate)
Pycnogel (pinus maritime)
Red clover (trifolium pretense)
St John's wort (hypericum perforatum)
Valerian (valeriana oficinalis)

Supplements

Supplements, including vitamins, minerals, amino acids and hormones, have become a regular part of many people's daily routines. Although no supplement can actually "cure" or "heal" epilepsy, some may be recommended by your doctor to alleviate the side effects of certain AEDs or treat certain conditions that could precipitate seizures.

However, before you ingest anything new (even something considered "natural" and "safe"), always consult your doctor and *never* stop taking your anti-seizure medications without your doctor's okay. Also, be aware that some supplements have the potential to interfere with your seizure medication or even provoke seizures.

Following is a list of some supplements that are related to epilepsy and seizures.

Vitamins

- *Vitamin B1 (thiamin)*
  Vitamin B1 deficiency could be associated with neurological problems and seizures.

- *Vitamin B6*
  A deficiency of this vitamin can cause seizures in newborns and infants that are reversed by the use of vitamin B6. It could rarely have the same effect in adults. It is also

frequently used in patients taking Levetiracetam (Keppra®) to prevent behavioral side effects

- *Vitamin B12*
  Vitamin B12 could be depleted by the use of some anti-epileptic medications (e. g. Dilantin). It has been reported that low levels of Vitamin B12 could lead to many neurological problems including seizures and mental inefficiency.

- *Folic acid*
  There are reports that a deficiency of folic acid, a member of the B-vitamin family, is associated with seizures, however, there is no clear proof. However there is proof that certain AEDs deplete the body of folic acid, like for example phenytoin (Dilantin®) so women of childbearing age must take supplements to help prevent birth defects related folic acid deficiency and the recommended dose ranges from 1-4 mg /day.

- *Vitamin D*
  Vitamin D deficiency could be seen in patients taking AEDs (e.g. Dilantin®, Phenobarbital). Since vitamin D is necessary for calcium metabolism, too little D can result in poor bone formation and/or osteoporosis. Supplements may be necessary if your doctor suspects a deficiency.

- *Vitamin E*
  There are reports that vitamin E supplements may help in children with intractable epilepsy, although more studies need to be done to confirm this. Vitamin E levels may be decreased by the use of some AEDs.

- *Vitamin K*
  Some AEDs (e.g. Dilantin®) could be associated with vitamin K deficiency. Vitamin K is essential for blood clotting so a deficiency could result in bleeding

Minerals

- *Calcium*
  Low calcium levels have the potential to bring on seizures and can also contribute to osteoporosis (thinning of the bones). Calcium deficiency may also be related to the use of some AEDs that either lower the levels of vitamin D or calcium levels or spur the liver to eliminate them faster (i.e. Dilantin®, Phenobarbital) Kidney problems, hormonal changes and alcohol abuse can contribute to deficiency of calcium and vitamin D.

- *Magnesium*
  Low magnesium levels can potentially cause seizures. Magnesium levels can be adversely affected by alcohol abuse, lack of magnesium intake and low calcium levels.

- *Manganese*
  Low Manganese has been reported to cause seizures, although this connection has not been clearly proven.

- *Selenium*
  There are reports (but no definitive proof) that a deficiency of Selenium is associated with seizures. Selenium supplements are sometime prescribed for patients taking valproic acid (Depakote®).

- *Sodium*
  Low Sodium is reported to have the potential to cause seizures as well as sleepiness and confusion. Low sodium can sometimes be a side effect of some AEDs (tegretol® and trileptal®). No supplements of sodium are necessary in general. Your doctor will probably have to reduce the amount of medication or even consider changing it if the sodium level does not come back to normal.

- *Zinc*

  Zinc is sometimes prescribed by the doctor in patients who are experiencing hair loss that is believed to be associated to the use of valproic acid (Depakote®)

Amino Acids

- *Carnitine*

  Carnitine is a derivative of the amino acid lysine. In patients taking certain anti-epileptic medications, valproic acid (Depakote®) in particular, there may be a deficit in Carnitine. Liver toxicity related to the use of valproic acid (Depakote®) has been related (but nor proven) to Carnitine deficiency. For this reason, sometimes your doctor will prescribe Carnitine supplements in patients taking valproic acid

- *Taurine*

  A deficiency in this has been linked to an increase in seizures, however there is no definitive proof of it.

Hormones

- *Melatonin*

  Melatonin is a hormone produced by the pineal gland. There is controversy whether Melatonin improves or worsens seizures. It is also used as a sleeping aid

Other CAM Therapies

Biofeedback, acupressure, yoga, tai-chi, massage and many others are among the CAM therapies that are sometimes tried to prevent future seizures, reduce stress or relieve other epilepsy-related problems. But like herbal therapy, they have not been subjected to enough scientific study to determine if they have a proven impact. However, the potential harm caused by these therapies is quite low, so they can usually be used safely along with traditional treatments for epilepsy. Still, check with your doctor before you try any therapies, especially any newer or unusual CAM, such as a more vigorous type of massage or yoga combined with extreme heat or intense breathing.

Increasing Relaxation and/or Relieving Stress

Since stress increases a propensity toward seizures, it makes sense that reducing stress and increasing relaxation could help with seizures. However, these methods do not have a directly proven effect on seizures. Therefore they should *not* replace your medical treatment and should only be used as a complementary therapy.

The advantages: they are mostly safe (but talk to your doctor before engaging in any of these therapies) and make you feel good. The disadvantages: they may be expensive and some are time-consuming.

- *Aromatherapy*
  This technique uses the aroma of plants and essential oils to produce relaxation and positive emotional changes. There are many different kinds of "aromas", some mild to some very strong.
  Jasmine has been proposed as a helpful for seizure control. There are some forms of aromatherapy that have been reported to worsen seizures and should be avoided. They include:
    - Camphor (Cinnamomum camphora)
    - Eucalyptus (Eucaliptus globulus)
    - Fennel (Foeniculum vulgare)
    - Hyssop (Hyssopus)
    - Pennyroyal Mentha pulegium)
    - Rosemary (Rosmarinus officinalis)
    - Sage (Salvia officinalis)
    - Savin (Juniperus sabina)
    - Spike lavender (Lavandula latifolia)
    - Tansy (tanacetum vulgare)
    - Thuja (thuya occidentalis)
    - Turpentine (Pinus species)
    - Wormwood (Artemisia absinthium)

Aromatherapy is provided by certified or registered aromatherapists.

- *Autogenic training*
  A relaxation technique somewhat like self-hypnosis, auto-genic training consists of brief sessions (about 20 minutes long) in which the person combines visual imagination, proper breathing techniques and self-instructions that are relaxing. Examples of self instructions include, "My left arm feels heavy", "I am in a warm bath completely relaxed,", and so on. There are also self-instructions to help you "come back" after relaxation, as in, "Now my left arm feels normal again and I am awake and at peace." It is recommended that this technique should be practiced daily in a comfortable and peaceful setting.

- *Massage*
  Massage involves the stroking and manipulation of the muscles and connective tissue in order to produce relaxation, relieve muscle tension and promote stress reduction. Rough massages should be avoided. Craniosacral therapy and chiropractic manipulations should be carefully discussed with your doctor in advance, and avoided if you have had brain surgery.

- *Meditation*
  This ancient practice is designed to increase self-awareness, reduce stress and help the individual experience the "present moment" through breathing techniques and the clearing of the mind of any stray thoughts. Nonjudgmental attitudes, gratitude and peacefulness are often reported results. It has been proposed as useful in increasing relaxation and second-arily, reducing the potential for seizures.

- *Music Therapy*
  This form of therapy is based on the theory that exposure to selections of music that have varying sequences of high and low tones can affect brain waves and physical reactions in the

body and the brain. Although it is undeniable that different melodies can bring forth certain feelings, there is no firm evidence that music can reduce seizure activity.

- *Neurofeedback*
Neurofeedback involves the recognition of "bad" brain waves on the EEG, and the use of techniques to help "correct" them and regulate stress. However, it is controversial whether or not this helps to control seizures.

- *Progressive Muscle Relaxation*
This method of producing relaxation and relieving stress involves the sequential tensing and relaxing of different muscles. After consciously contracting a set of muscles, the relaxation that follows is deeper than usual and can help relax the entire body. This is therefore proposed as possibly beneficial in seizure reduction although there is no direct evidence of this.

- *Yoga*
This method, which unifies the actions and intentions of the body, mind and heart, involves a combination of unique body positions and conscious breathing exercises. Yoga is well known for its relaxing, stress-relieving properties. There have been studies in the last few years to determine whether it can affect seizure frequency; results are still inconclusive. There are many variants of yoga including some more novel and unusual types (i.e. laughing yoga, hot yoga). As always, consult with your doctor before engaging in this form of exercise.

Non-Traditional Medicine

Non-traditional forms of medicine may be able to provide an alternative to patients who do not respond to conventional therapy. However they do not have any directly proven positive effects on seizures, and there is always the danger of unintended consequences and adverse events. Therefore, they should never replace your medical treatment and you must always consult your doctor before engaging in any of these therapies. And even if your doctor approves, these should only be used as complementary therapies.

- *Acupuncture*
  This technique, which involves the insertion of needles into specific points on the body, is based on the idea that the body contains an energy flow called "qi" and that symptoms of disease arise when this energy is blocked. The insertion of needles is believed to unblock the energy flow and allow the body to heal itself. Supporting evidence as regards to seizure control is not available.

- *Homeopathy*
  The theory behind homeopathy is that exposure to a small amount of a preparation that produces the same symptoms already affecting the patient will stimulate healing processes in the body. Preparations can include extracts from plants, minerals and even human or animal tissue. Supporting evidence as regards to seizure control is not available.

- *Hyperbaric Oxygen Therapy*
  During this treatment, the patient breathes 100% oxygen while under increased atmospheric pressure. Reports are contradictory as to whether this form of treatment can help in treating autism or epilepsy and there is no solid evidence for this.

- *Neuropathic Medicine*
  Neuropathic medicine combines standard Western medicine with therapeutic diets and preventive approaches. Neuropaths are licensed primary health care providers (as opposed to homeopaths who are not.). Although this form

of medicine presents interesting possibilities much more research is needed.

- *Traditional Chinese medicine*
  Those who specialize in this ancient form of medicine combine Chinese herbs, diets and acupuncture to treat many different medical conditions. Again, although this form of medicine is highly interesting, more research is still needed.

Tell Your Doctor Everything!

Experimenting with CAM treatments such as herbal therapies without informing your doctor could create major problems. Even "natural" therapies affect body chemistry and may make seizure medication less effective.

For these reasons, find a doctor well-versed in epilepsy who will work with you and can openly discuss the benefits and risks of CAM treatments. Yoga, meditation, and biofeedback have minimal risks, and if they make you feel better, there is usually little to no downside. For some, supportive treatments such as psychotherapy might be the best treatment option, perhaps in conjunction with antidepressants or other medication. And don't forget the immense importance of a good diet, plenty of sleep and regular exercise, as these are the foundation for good health.

Recognizing/Preventing Seizures or Monitoring Seizures That Do Occur

If you know that a seizure is about to occur, you may be able to take steps to prevent it by taking medication, relaxing and removing yourself from a stressful situation and/or get to a safe place before the seizure ensues. A seizure alert dog may be able to warn you that a seizure is about to happen:

- *Seizure Alert Dogs*
  These service dogs are reportedly able to warn you of a seizure that is coming minutes or even hours before it happens. It is

not really clear how these dogs "know" this, but they often play an essential role in making sure their owners are in a safe position before the seizure strikes and in keeping them safe both during and after the seizure.

While the following devices won't warn you that a seizure is about to happen, they may be able to record the occurrence of a seizure, collect data during a seizure and alert caretakers.

- *Movement Monitors*
  Mattress pads and alarms worn as wristwatches can alert caretakers about the occurrence of an unwitnessed seizure. Most of these are still being researched to determine whether they are really reliable seizure detectors and are not yet FDA approved.

- *Oxygen monitors*
  These are usually attached to a finger and monitor both heart rate and blood oxygenation which would change during a seizure.

- *Baby monitors*
  A less technologically-advanced yet inventive way some caretakers have come up with to monitor a patient for seizures in another room is to set up a baby monitor. The noise produced by the patient will alert the caretaker (even if he or she is asleep), who may be able to help the patient avoid injury.

The Final Word on CAM – So Far

While we're not sure whether CAM is truly effective in reducing the frequency or severity of seizures, we do know that certain forms (e.g. massage, meditation, progressive relaxation, yoga) can help relieve stress, anxiety, depression, headaches and other problems stemming from epilepsy. Thus, as long you keep your doctor fully informed about the CAM you're using (or even considering), and your doctor has investigated and found it's not harmful, CAM may be a helpful adjunct treatment.

CHAPTER TEN
LIVING WITH EPILEPSY – SPECIAL MEDICAL TOPICS

Epilepsy, like all disorders, affects people in different ways and causes problems that may seem completely unrelated to the occurrence of seizures. Thus, even if your seizures are under excellent control, you can experience challenges that may stem from the disorder itself, the medications you are taking or epilepsy-related mood changes.

Drug side effects can be controlled, if not eliminated, by a change in medication and/or dosage. Other difficulties may recede or disappear simply because you follow the rules of good health: eat properly, get enough sleep, get plenty of exercise, take medication as prescribed, and see your doctor regularly for treatment protocol evaluation.

It also pays to be aware of certain problems that can crop up so you will be better prepared to handle them. In this chapter, we'll look at the epilepsy-related issues common to certain groups, specifically men, women and the elderly, and the emotional problems and memory/cognitive difficulties that may accompany the disorder. The most important thing to remember is that almost *all* of these problems are controllable.

MEN'S ISSUES

Epilepsy does not play favorites, striking males and females alike. Yet there are a few differences in incidence and side effects. Men, for example, are more likely to develop post-traumatic epilepsy because they tend to engage in physically dangerous activities more often than women do. And men can develop certain sexual problems that don't affect women because their sexual "equipment" is so different.

Although the majority of men with epilepsy are able to enjoy a healthy sex life, the seizures and anti-seizure medications can have unwanted effects on sexual health and performance. Specifically, the sex drive may diminish, sexual performance may be impaired, and psychological issues can arise (such as the fear of having a seizure during sex) that put a damper on sexual relations. In addition, fertility rates are slightly decreased in men with epilepsy due to lower sperm counts, abnormally shaped sperm, and low sperm motility, although most men with epilepsy are able to father children.

Generally, epilepsy-related sexual problems can be broken down into two categories: physical and medication side effects.

Physical

Arousal and intimacy are complex phenomena that require a great deal of brain activity, both subtle and obvious. Seizures can interfere with portions of the brain that control sexual desire and performance and/or alter the delicate hormonal balance required for a healthy sex life. Fortunately, sexual health is often restored through hormonal treatments. For example, testosterone replacement can help restore a man's libido and may also be helpful in relieving a depressed mood.

Medication Side Effects

Certain medications such as phenytoin (Dilantin®) and carbamazepine (Tegretol®, Carbatrol®) can alter the actions of various hormones, resulting in a decrease in sexual desire and performance. Older seizure medications, such as phenobarbital (Luminal®) and primidone (Mysoline®), can make it difficult to achieve an erection due to their effects on male hormones. Men taking phenytoin (Dilantin®)

or phenobarbital (Luminal®) may also develop Peyronie's disease, which produces a painful, curved erection. (Although this problem has been associated with these medicines, it has not been definitively proven that they cause this condition). The good news is that these side effects typically disappear when medications are changed.

Although epilepsy may cause sexual problems for some men, the majority experience healthy sex lives and are able to become fathers. While it can be difficult to discuss problems like a decreased sex drive or impotence with your doctor, it is worth the   discomfort. These symptoms often result from medication, so changes in treatment may make them go away. If a different medical issue is the culprit, a visit to an endocrinologist or fertility specialist might be necessary for further testing and treatment. But take heart – the outcome is good in most cases!

WOMEN'S ISSUES

Like men, women with epilepsy can face a declining interest in sex, difficulty with sexual function and fertility problems. They must also wrestle with challenges involving pregnancy, menstruation, birth control and other issues. The epilepsy-related problems that belong strictly to women include seizures that occur at a certain point in the menstrual cycle, polycystic ovary syndrome and early menopause. Osteoporosis is more prevalent but not exclusive of women. Because each of these problems is quite complex, we'll need to take a look at them one by one.

Catamenial Epilepsy: "Women's Seizures"

About one-third of women with epilepsy develop hormone-sensitive seizures at certain points in the menstrual cycle, a condition called *catamenial epilepsy*. The menstrual cycle itself is not to blame, yet the causes of catamenial epilepsy are still not well understood. They may include any of the following:

- Fluctuations in the levels of estrogen and progesterone

- Changes in the amount of bodily fluid and electrolytes (e.g. sodium and other blood compounds)

- Psychological stress

- Variations in the levels of antiseizure medications in the body (this is related to hormonal changes)

Of these four causes, the most important may be the changes in female hormone levels that occur throughout the monthly cycle. The proportions of estrogen and progesterone change constantly. To illustrate, if you consider Day 1 of the cycle to be the first day of the menstrual period, the estrogen levels will be higher during the first 14 days, while progesterone levels during this time will be almost non-existent. Then at Day 14 they switch, with estrogen falling and leveling out while progesterone rises and becomes the dominant hormone. Both hormones drop off at Day 28, a phenomenon that triggers the next menstrual period.

How does all of this rising and falling and switching from estrogen dominance to progesterone dominance affect epileptic seizures? The answer is fairly simple: Estrogen favors seizures while progesterone protects against them. This means that seizures are more likely to occur when the level of estrogen is high or the level of progesterone is low, in relation to each other. These situations occur:

- Just before ovulation in the middle of the cycle, when estrogen levels peak

- Just before the onset of the menstrual period, when progesterone levels suddenly drop

- During a menstrual cycle when there is no egg released, which means no progesterone is produced. That's because progesterone is created by the "casing" that houses the egg. Once the egg pops out of its "house," that casing becomes a progesterone-producing factory. But if no egg is produced (a phenomenon known as an "anovulatory cycle"), there is no casing and, thus, no production of progesterone. Women with epilepsy tend to have more anovulatory cycles than average. And seizures tend to occur during the second half of an anovulatory cycle (Day 14 – 28), when progesterone levels would normally increase.

If you have or suspect that you have catamenial epilepsy, keep a diary of your menstrual periods and your seizures to see if there is a pattern and discuss the possibility with your doctor. He or she may respond by giving you reproductive hormones/natural progesterone, or increasing your dosage of antiseizure medications during a particular phase of your menstrual cycle. The medicine acetazolamide (Diamox®), a gentle diuretic with some mild anti-seizure effects, has also been shown to help in some patients.

Epilepsy, Fertility and Polycystic Ovary Syndrome

Research has shown that women with epilepsy have fewer children, which may be due to sexual dysfunction, more frequent anovulatory menstrual cycles, fear of producing a child with a birth defect or other factors.

One of those other factors may be polycystic ovary syndrome (PCOS), a condition in which imbalanced female sex hormones produce ovarian cysts, alterations in the menstrual cycle, difficulty in becoming pregnant and other problems. By definition, a woman with PCOS has two of the following three symptoms:

- Multiple cysts in the ovaries

- High levels of male hormone

- Excessive facial hair and acne

And there may be other symptoms such as obesity, irregular menstrual periods or frequent anovulatory cycles. Although any woman can develop polycystic ovary syndrome, it is twice as common in women with epilepsy, possibly because seizure activity in the brain alters the production of hormones. The medicine valproic acid (Depakote®), which is used for seizures and other disorders, can cause symptoms similar to those seen in polycystic ovary syndrome. If you notice any of these symptoms, see your neurologist, gynecologist or an endocrinologist.

Birth Control Pills vs. Antiseizure Medications

While some women with epilepsy find it difficult to become pregnant, others may suddenly find themselves expecting an unplanned baby arrival. Be aware that certain antiseizure medications decrease the effectiveness of birth control pills and other forms of hormonal birth control (e.g. hormones implanted into body tissue, injected under the skin, absorbed from a patch on the skin, or placed in the vagina). The main AEDs that can cause birth control failure include:

- carbamazepine (Tegretol®, Carbatrol®)

- felbamate (Felbatol®)

- oxcarbazepine (Trileptal®)

- phenytoin (Dilantin®)

- rufinamide (Banzel®)

- topiramate (Topamax®)

If you are taking birth control pills or using other forms of hormonal birth control, talk with your epileptologist and your gynecologist to determine the best combination of antiseizure medication and birth control methods. Possible solutions include AEDs that do not interact with birth control pills, and alternative birth control methods (i.e. condoms). Birth control pills containing a higher dose of estrogen are sometimes recommended, although they might not provide adequate contraception and could contribute to an increase in seizure frequency.

Just as AEDs can interfere with birth control, birth control pills may interfere with the effectiveness of certain antiseizure medicines. For example, blood levels of lamotrigine (Lamictal®) can be decreased by birth control pills, resulting in poor seizure control. If you have epilepsy and are taking birth control pills, be sure that your gynecologist and epileptologist are both aware of the situation and can adjust your medication types and dosages accordingly.

Epilepsy and Menopause
Women with epilepsy typically experience menopause earlier than expected, possibly due to the effects of seizures on areas of the brain that regulate reproductive hormones. During perimenopause, the several-year transitional period that culminates in the complete absence of menstrual periods, some women experience an increase in seizure frequency, especially those with catamenial epilepsy. This could be explained by the increase of estrogen in relation to progesterone that occurs during perimenopause. Estrogen, as you will remember, promotes seizures, while progesterone protects against them. The increase in seizures may also be related to other perimenopausal symptoms such as hot flashes or insomnia.

The effect of the postmenopausal period on seizure frequency is unclear. There may be fewer seizures, especially in those with catamenial epilepsy, because of lower estrogen levels. But in those who use hormone replacement therapy that includes estrogen, there may be an increase in seizure frequency. If the symptoms of perimenopause/

menopause are too uncomfortable, some experts recommend carefully monitored treatment with a single estrogen and natural progesterone. And for any woman with epilepsy going through perimenopause or menopause, AED medication adjustments may be necessary due to the changes in hormone levels.

Epilepsy and Osteoporosis

Osteoporosis, the thinning and weakening of the bones, is seen more commonly in postmenopausal women and can lead to bone fractures. Risk factors include eating disorders, being very thin, tobacco use, consumption of excessive amounts of alcohol, low calcium intake, taking corticosteroid medicines and certain other medications, being white or Asian and/or having a family history of osteoporosis.

If the disease is severe enough, it can trigger fractures that occur spontaneously, without a fall or other injury. It's actually possible for a weight-bearing bone to break when you're just standing or walking normally! Taking certain antiseizure medications, including carbamazepine (Tegretol®, Carbatro®)), phenobarbital (Luminal®), phenytoin (Dilantin®) and primidone (Mysoline®), can increase the likelihood of developing osteoporosis and should be avoided by those at risk of this disease. If you have osteoporosis, thinning of the bones or any risk factors for the disease, be sure to tell your doctor, who will make changes to your AEDs accordingly.

Besides avoiding medicines that increase the risk of osteoporosis, it pays to take other steps to protect your bones. Preventive measures include getting regular, weight-bearing exercise; consuming a balanced diet; avoiding alcohol, caffeine and smoking; and taking calcium and vitamin D supplements.

EPILEPSY AND SLEEP

Although sleep troubles can plague just about anybody, women and the elderly seem especially vulnerable. Insomnia can be a very serious problem for those with epilepsy, as getting too little sleep can provoke seizures. Yet, ironically, AEDs themselves can sometimes disturb sleep and, as a result, facilitate seizures. Epilepsy is also associated with anxiety, which can promote sleeplessness, which can cause seizures. It's a vicious circle.

How much sleep do you need? While there is no magic number of hours that will prevent seizures, most adults require 7 to 8 hours per night. Children and infants, of course, will require more. Rearrange your schedule, make sure your nighttime environment is conducive to sleeping, and do whatever else you can to ensure you get plenty of sleep on a nightly basis.

If you have trouble falling asleep and/or staying asleep, try adopting these good sleep hygiene tips:

- Don't eat too much prior to bedtime, as digestion can interfere with sleep.

- Don't exercise too close to bedtime. Your body shifts into high gear when exercising and takes awhile to calm down, making it hard to drift off too soon after exercising.

- Before bedtime avoid mental stimulation, as in spellbinding books, TV shows or computer activities or anything else that might interfere with falling asleep.

- Try to go to bed at the same time each night; get up at the same time each morning. Your body will appreciate the regularity.

- Avoid caffeinated products such as coffee, soda and chocolates any time after 12 noon, as they can over-stimulate the brain, even hours later causing insomnia.

- If you are not asleep 20-30 minutes after going to bed, get out of bed and go into another room to read or do something boring and routine like folding laundry. Wait until you feel sleepy again before you get back into bed. Your body will start to associate bed with sleeping rather than with wakefulness.

- Some seizure medications, such as lamotrigine (Lamictal®), cause insomnia. Ask your doctor about taking the bulk of the dosage earlier in the day or changing your medication.

- Other seizure medications, like phenobarbital (Luminal®) and clonazepam (Klonopin®), can cause drowsiness during the day. Try taking the bulk of the dosage at bedtime.

- Sleep apnea (brief pauses in breathing during sleep) is more common in people with epilepsy than in the general population. If you feel sleepy during the day and are overweight, snore or have facial deformities, consider getting tested for sleep apnea by a sleep specialist. Untreated sleep apnea can lead to seizures, high blood pressure and other medical problems.

- Disturbed sleep may be a symptom of anxiety or depression, which can be treated successfully when recognized and addressed. Ask your doctor for a referral to a psychiatrist or psychologist for an evaluation.

- Seizures themselves can interfere with sleep. If you wake up with muscle soreness, tongue bites or a wet bed, you may be having seizures during sleep. Sometimes overnight EEG tests can detect seizure activity while you are asleep.

My patients often ask me if it's all right to take "sleeping pills." While they are not inherently bad, the sleep produced by sleeping aids is not as restful as natural sleep. And, of course, dependence might develop. Before taking one, you should be evaluated for underlying causes of your sleep disturbance. Then, if your doctor thinks a sleeping aid is necessary, certain commonly used medications such as zolpidem (Ambien®) don't appear to have a negative impact on epilepsy. Melatonin, a supplement often used for insomnia, is probably safe for people with epilepsy, although it has not been studied extensively.

Be aware that caution should be used when combining sleeping medication with certain seizure medications such as phenobarbital (Luminal®) or benzodiazepines (e.g. Klonopin® or Valium®), as the combination could result in excessive sedation.

THE SPECIAL PROBLEMS OF THE ELDERLY

Epilepsy is very common in the elderly; thus, the number of people who have the disorder will rise as the Baby Boomers move into their golden years. Although the underlying mechanisms of seizures do not change with advancing age, their harmful effects on general health and quality of life may be increased.

Epilepsy that develops later in life tends to be partial-onset rather than generalized onset and is usually acquired (often due to strokes) rather than inherited (due to genetic causes). The most common causes of epilepsy in seniors are cerebrovascular disease (strokes and brain bleeds) and brain tumors. Falls are also a causative factor, as they can rupture the fragile blood vessels in the elderly brain, leaving scar tissue that may become a seizure focus. There is also a small increase in the risk of epilepsy in people who have Alzheimer's disease, Parkinson's, or are chronic alcohol abusers. Epilepsy in a senior may also mark the return of a seizure disorder that was in remission, or could be a continuation of a lifelong problem.

Diagnosis in the Elderly

Diagnosing epilepsy in the elderly tends to be more challenging than it is in younger people for several reasons:

- The elderly are more likely to have smaller, more subtle seizures, such as episodes of blank staring, as opposed to dramatic tonic-clonic seizures. These staring episodes can easily be dismissed by the elderly person or the caretaker as "senior moments."

- Because the elderly are more likely to live alone or be socially isolated, the seizures may not be seen by others. Or it could be that an elderly partner has witnessed a seizure, but is unable to remember or describe it.

- Elderly people with dementia, stroke, developmental delay or autism may find it difficult to impossible to describe seizure symptoms to their doctors or caretakers.

Unfortunately, an unwarranted diagnosis of epilepsy in the elderly is common. It may be blamed for confusion or a loss of consciousness that is actually due to other medical conditions, such as infections or heart disease. And the common practice of over-prescribing seizure medications, especially prevalent in nursing homes, can cause serious problems including medication toxicity, drug interactions, bone loss, depression, sedation, liver damage, rash and fever, just to name a few.

Treatment in the Elderly

Leaping over the hurdle of correct diagnosis is just the beginning, as the treatment of *any* medical problem in the elderly requires special care. Senior citizens may have poorer health overall, other diseases/disorders that can complicate the issue, and altered metabolisms and other physiologic issues that must be taken into consideration. For example, as the metabolism slows with age, the ability to "process" and eliminate medications weakens, which may allow levels of medication and metabolic byproducts to rise. This can trigger side effects or an overdose in the elderly, even when they are taking the "standard" amount.

Not only does the metabolism slow with advancing age, the ability to absorb medications changes – sometimes from day to day. This means that on some days a good portion of the dosage may be absorbed, while on others only a small percentage is absorbed, causing fluctuations in the blood levels of the medication.

There is also a big problem with drug interaction. Most elderly individuals take two to three medications daily, while 20 percent take more than five medications to manage a variety of medical conditions. Many commonly used medications share the same metabolic pathways in the liver as the AEDS, so one may raise or lower the levels of the other. For example, carbamazepine (Tegretol®, Carbatrol®) lowers levels of the blood thinner warfarin (Coumadin®), a medication that helps prevent blood clots and strokes. Since both seizures and strokes are serious medical issues, you can't simply drop one medication. Instead, a delicate balance must be achieved.

The elderly are also more prone to side effects caused by seizure medications. The toll taken by side effects is directly related to the number of medications taken. For example, an elderly person who already struggles with balance issues will be more likely to fall if he or she takes many different medications. Falls are particularly dangerous as they can result in fractures of fragile bones or serious head injuries. The result can be seizures, prolonged and costly hospitalization, or even death.

Further complicating matters is the increased incidence of memory loss seen in this age group, making them more likely to take their medications incorrectly and/or miss doses. A pillbox can help keep the elderly person organized, and an alarm clock can serve as a reminder that it's time to take the medication. When possible, extended-release forms of medication can eliminate the need for multiple daily dosages.

Medication on a Budget

It's a tough choice when you're forced to choose between eating and paying the rent or buying your medications. Fortunately, Patient Assistance Programs offer free or low cost medications to those who can't afford them. See http://www.rxassist.org/ for a comprehensive directory of Patient Assistance Programs.

Proper Medical Care of the Elderly

For the reasons mentioned above, it is vital that the diagnosis be correct. All the appropriate tests should be performed including, if indicated, a video-EEG to capture and classify spells. Once the diagnosis of epilepsy has been made, the proper medication should be selected. Medications such as lamotrigine (Lamictal®) and leviteracitam (Keppra®) have been shown to be safe and effective in the elderly, with fewer side effects than the older seizure medications, such as carbamazepine (Tegretol®, Carbatrol®). However, only the *minimum* dose and *minimum* number of seizure medications should be prescribed. Blood work should be done regularly to check medication levels and other factors.

A careful record should be kept of any side effects experienced. (This may require the assistance of family members and caregivers.) This will help the doctor decide whether to increase/decrease the dosage or substitute a completely different medication, in order to minimize unwanted effects. Should surgery be an option, rest assured that it has been shown to be safe and effective in the elderly. Still, it should only be considered for those who fail to respond to conventional medical treatment.

Finally, the treatment regimen should be reviewed and updated regularly, as evolving needs require changes in treatment. Even those who have had well-controlled epilepsy for a long time should have their treatment protocol reviewed by an epileptologist or neurologist once they reach the age of 65 or 70.

EMOTIONAL PROBLEMS AND EPILEPSY

As if physical problems weren't enough, about half of all people with epilepsy are troubled by depression or anxiety. It's a sad fact that those with epilepsy are about five to ten times more likely to commit suicide than those in the general population. Fortunately, there are now many treatment options for depression and anxiety, and about 80% of those who are treated will improve. Before treatment can be started, however, someone will have to notice that the person is suffering.

Common signs of depression include:

- Feeling blue most of the time

- Becoming much less interested in activities once enjoyed

- A weight gain or weight loss over the course of a month (not because of dieting)

- Sleeping too much or not being able to sleep

- Feeling very tired

- Feeling sluggish, or overly-active and fidgety

- Feeling guilty for unwarranted reasons

- A feeling of being "less" than most other people

- Having trouble concentrating

- Experiencing reduced sexual desire

- Having suicidal thoughts (If this is stated by a loved one, it must always be taken seriously and discussed immediately with the doctor!)

Common signs of anxiety include:

- Free-floating nervousness and feelings of being unsettled during most of the day (In epilepsy, this may be linked to wondering if and when a seizure will occur.)

- Poor sleep

- Poor concentration

- Rapid heart rate

- Jitteriness

- Feeling choked up and having trouble breathing

- Worrying about bad things happening in the future

- Sweating when it is not hot or blushing

- Poor appetite or digestive problems

If you recognize any of these signs of depression or anxiety in yourself (or, if you are a caregiver or family member, in the person who has epilepsy), talk it over with your doctor. He or she may refer you to a specialist (either a psychiatrist or psychologist) for evaluation and possible treatment. It's important to remember that suicidal thoughts are considered a psychiatric emergency and professional help must be sought right away.

MEMORY, THINKING SKILLS AND EPILEPSY

Epilepsy commonly affects memory and thinking, sometimes significantly. Memory problems can range from having difficulty recalling where you put your keys to keeping track of meetings or appointments. There can be difficulty with word finding ("I know what I want to say, but just can't seem to come up with the right word"), comprehending language ("I have trouble understanding what I've read") and sustaining attention ("I find myself zoning out when watching TV or having a conversation with a friend").

Why Does Epilepsy Affect Memory and Thinking?

You may be wondering what memory has to do with epilepsy. The connection between epilepsy and memory problems can be explained by the *Quadruple Whammy Effect:*

- Electrical activity in the brain during or between seizures can disrupt thinking and memory.

- Memory can be disturbed if the seizure focus is near "memory centers."

- Medications can have side effects that disrupt thinking and memory.

- Depression and anxiety, which frequently accompany epilepsy, can upset thinking and memory.

Of course, not all memory problems can be blamed on epilepsy; sometimes the real culprit is a disease like dementia or simple aging. If you're experiencing memory problems and wondering if they are related to your epilepsy, a neuropsychologist (a Ph.D. or Psy.D. with specialized training in the testing of brain functions) can assess your memory and other thinking skills, such as attention and language. Your different types of memory (yes, there are several) will be measured and compared to others in your age group.

The tests involved are not painful and require answering questions, copying drawings and putting together designs with blocks. While there are several hours of testing involved and you may end up feeling exhausted, the results can be valuable and lead to important changes in your treatment.

Once testing is completed, your results will be compared to the "norms." This information will be combined with your medical history and other records to determine the source of any problems.

Examples of changes in your treatment that could occur because of test results include:

- Discontinuing medications that could be affecting your thinking, and substituting others that don't have this effect.

- A referral to a psychologist/psychiatrist for treatment of emotional problems that may be interfering with your thinking and learning processes.

- A letter addressed to your work or school asking for certain accommodations such as a quiet environment for you to work in, extra time for test taking, a person who can take notes for you, a teacher that repeats instructions a few times and so on.

- A referral to a memory treatment program.

All of these recommendations can be very helpful when they target your specific problem.

Can Treatment Restore My Memory?

Memory treatment cannot bring your memory back, but it can improve your mental efficiency. Most memory treatment programs begin with an explanation of how your memory works and how epilepsy plays a role in undermining it. Next, they help you discover and understand your mental strengths and weaknesses so you can begin to rely more on the strengths. Then you'll learn techniques that can help you compensate for your memory weaknesses, and you'll be given opportunities to implement these techniques. Finally, you will learn ways to improve your attention, planning, organization and time management skills.

Do Alzheimer's Drugs Help?

Many patients have asked me if the medicines used to treat memory loss in Alzheimer's disease, such as galantamine (Razadyne®) or donepezil (Aricept®), can combat the memory loss seen in epilepsy. Unfortunately, relatively few group studies on this topic have been conducted and individual case studies do not seem to be showing much success. However, more research is needed to answer this question fully.

LIVING THE GOOD LIFE

Never lose sight that it is possible to live a normal, happy life when you have epilepsy. Like with many other challenges that life throws your way you'll probably need to make certain adjustments. By working closely with your doctor, following the principles of healthy living, taking your medications as prescribed, paying attention to your body's signals and utilizing various adjunct treatment programs when necessary, you *can* achieve and maintain a state of physical, mental and emotional balance. And it can last a lifetime.

CHAPTER ELEVEN
PREGNANCY – BEFORE, DURING AND AFTER

—————————————— ● ——————————————

If you're one of the one million American women of childbearing age who has epilepsy, you're probably wondering if it's safe to get pregnant. And thanks to new knowledge and better access to early, regular prenatal care, the answer is *yes* – most women with epilepsy will be able to experience normal pregnancies without complications. In fact, currently over 90% of babies born to women with epilepsy are healthy! However, certain problems do occur more frequently in pregnant women with epilepsy and their babies, making it imperative that you become well-informed and take certain steps before you take this important step in life. Then, if you do decide you want to conceive and carry a child, you must be closely monitored by your obstetrician and neurologist/epileptologist *from pre-conception onward*.

COMPLICATIONS THAT *MAY* OCCUR

Although your chances of delivering a healthy baby are excellent, there *is* an increased risk that you'll experience certain pregnancy complications. And there is a greater likelihood that various physical or mental problems may affect your baby. Let's start with what you, yourself, might face during pregnancy.

Health Problems in the Mother
If you have epilepsy, you are more likely to experience one or more of the following complications. (Antiseizure medications appear to contribute to some of these problems.)

- **Frequent nausea** – Besides being unpleasant, increased nausea and/or vomiting can make it difficult or impossible to take or retain a sufficient dosage of AEDs for seizure prevention.

- **Vaginal bleeding during and after pregnancy**- This is more common in women using antiseizure medications.

- **Anemia**

- **Placental abruption** (early separation of the placenta from the uterus)

- **Pre-eclampsia** (high blood pressure and excessive protein in the urine) – Pre-eclampsia is twice as likely to occur in women with epilepsy, compared to women without epilepsy. It is also more common in those who are taking antiseizure medications.

- **Fetal death** – Defined as the loss of the baby after 20 weeks of gestation, fetal death occurs in mothers with epilepsy up to twice as often as in the general population. This may be due to due to congenital malformations .

- **Increase in seizure frequency** – Affecting about 15-30% of women, the increase in seizures is usually due to insufficient doses of medication, which can result from non-compliance, nausea and vomiting, and pregnancy-related changes in metabolism. Other non-medication causes include sleep deprivation, hormonal changes and the psychological/emotional stress of pregnancy.

Most of these can be prevented or successfully treated if they are detected early enough. But you must be vigilant. Immediately report any unusual symptoms you may experience (excessive fatigue, pain, nausea, bleeding, fainting) and certainly any seizures and make sure your obstetrician and epileptologist follow your progress closely. By becoming as well-informed as possible and working closely with your doctors, these risks can be reduced considerably.

Health Problems in the Baby

Unfortunately, the babies of women with epilepsy have an increased risk of suffering from various problems, some that are immediately apparent and others that may not surface until later. Problems that are readily apparent include birth defects, neonatal internal hemorrhaging (internal bleeding), and low birth weight/prematurity.

- **Birth defects** – Structural or functional abnormalities that cause physical or mental disabilities occur approximately twice as often in children of epileptic mothers, compared to the general population. Birth defects fall into one of two categories: minor malformations, which are those that do not affect the baby's overall health, and major malformations, which are those of surgical, medical and/or cosmetic importance.

    o *Minor malformations include:*
      unusual facial features
      finger abnormalities
      toe abnormalities

    o *Major malformations include:*
      Cleft lip or cleft palate
      Congenital heart defects
      Neural tube defects (spina bifida)
      Skeletal abnormalities
      Urinary tract defects

Cleft lip or cleft palate make up about 30 percent of the increased risk of malformations.

Most fetal malformations are associated with exposure to AEDs in utero. For this reason, medication adjustments should be made *before* conception. And during pregnancy, it's recommended that the minimal possible number of AED be taken, using the lowest possible dose that is still controlling seizures.

- **Neonatal hemorrhaging** – Characterized by uncontrolled internal bleeding in the infant, this disorder develops within 24 hours of delivery. The biggest concern is bleeding in the brain, which could cause permanent brain damage. Some of the AED's may interfere with vitamin K metabolism and therefore with vitamin K-dependent clotting factors. Fortunately, vitamin K injections are given routinely to all newborns at birth, and maternal supplementation with 10 mg vitamin K1 during the last month of pregnancy can usually prevent this problem. Historically, most women on AEDs received oral vitamin K supplementation during the last month of pregnancy. Recent studies raised some controversy about usefulness of this practice.

- **Low birth weight** – Low birth weight (weight of less than 2500g) is seen about twice as often in babies of epileptic mothers, whether or not AEDs were used during pregnancy. Seizures during pregnancy seem to be linked to low birth weight. There is also an increased risk of intrauterine growth retardation, in which the weight of the embryo, fetus or newborn is less than the 10th percentile of the predicted weight-for-age. Both conditions are more likely when the baby is exposed in utero to AEDs, especially when more than one of these medications is used.

Complications that can arise or become apparent weeks, months or years later include:

- **Developmental delay and/or learning disabilities** – Children of epileptic mothers are approximately twice as likely to experience developmental delay, which is defined as any significant lag in a child's physical, cognitive, emotional, behavioral or social development when compared to the norm. This was linked to numerous factors including number of seizures during pregnancy and exposure to AED's.

- **Increased risk of developing epilepsy** – The risk of a child of an epileptic mother developing epilepsy is about three times higher (3 percent) than the risk seen in the general population, but *only* if epilepsy occurs in the mother, not the father.

- **Reduced growth potential** – The intrauterine growth retardation and low birth weight seen during pregnancy and at birth may continue as a reduced growth potential, which can be seen in some children whether their mothers took AEDs during pregnancy or not.

You can decrease the chances of your baby suffering from these problems by getting proper medical care before and during pregnancy. As with maternal complications, early diagnosis of complications affecting the baby (even before birth) can be critical to the prevention of these problems and/or significantly improve the outcome.

TAKING ANTI-SEIZURE MEDICATIONS DURING PREGNANCY

It's very important that you retain seizure control during pregnancy. Generalized seizures can harm your baby by causing you to fall and injure yourself or the baby. The baby may become oxygen deprived, resulting in brain damage and developmental delay. Seizures during pregnancy are also associated with a greater likelihood of miscarriage and stillbirth, as well as an increased risk of epilepsy developing in the child.

Yet taking AEDs during pregnancy also presents risks. The primary concern is birth defects (see the major and minor malformations listed above) and cognitive impairment. Taking more than one AED or higher doses of an AED increases the danger. Thus, the risks of suffering seizures must be carefully balanced with the risks of taking medication.

Caution! *Do not change doses or stop taking medications without first discussing it with your epileptologist or neurologist.*

Assessing the Risk

The FDA has established certain guidelines concerning the effects and risks of medications on reproduction and pregnancy. These guidelines divide the medications into four groups (A, B, C and D). All AEDs belong to Category C and Category D, which are defined as follows:

Category C Anti-Seizure Medications

There is a lack of good human studies testing the effects of these medications during pregnancy. However, when pregnant animals were treated with some of these medicines, their babies had an increased risk of suffering from birth defects. Some medicines in this category have *not* been studied in either pregnant animals or humans, which means we can't say with certainty what effect(s) they might have. Regarding the medicines in this class, the FDA states that: *"In some situations the medicine may still help the mothers and babies more than it might harm."*

AEDs that fall into Category C include:

- ethosuximide (Zarontin®)

- felbamate (Felbatol®)

- gabapentin (Neurontin®)

- lacosamide (Vimpat®)

- lamotrigine (Lamictal®)

- levetiracetam (Keppra®)

- oxcarbazepine (Trileptal®)

- pregabalin (Lyrica®)

- rufinamide (Banzel®)

- tiagabine (Gabitril®)

- vigabatrin (Sabril®)

- zonisamide (Zonegran®)

Category D Anti-Seizure Medications

Studies in humans and other reports show that some pregnant women who used the medicines in this category *did* have babies that were born with problems related to the medicine. The FDA concludes that: *"In some situations, the medicine may still help the mother and the baby more than it might harm."*

AEDs that fall into Category D include:

- carbamazepine (Tegretol®, Carbatrol®)

- clonazepam (Klonopin®)

- diazepam (Valium®)

- lorazepam (Ativan®)

- phenobarbital (Luminal®)

- phenytoin (Dilantin®, Phenytek®)

- primidone (Mysoline®)

- topiramate (Topamax®)

- valproic acid (Depakote®)

The FDA pregnancy categories imply that category D medications are associated with higher risks than Category C. It is important to note that seizures in a pregnant woman can also be damaging to the unborn child. The risks due to seizures compared to the risks due to anti-seizure medications must be carefully balanced.

The North American Antiepileptic Drug Pregnancy Registry
United States and Canada established a Pregnancy Registry for the purposes of gathering very important information about the effects of antiseizure medications and epilepsy on pregnancy. You are invited to join the Registry and add to this valuable database. All information is confidential. Your participation would involve only three telephone interviews: at the time of enrollment, during the 7th month of your pregnancy, and few months after delivery.

If you'd like to participate, please see http://www2.massgeneral.org/aed/.
You can also call their toll free telephone number: 1-888-233-2334

BEFORE YOU GET PREGNANT...

Because your pregnancy will involve a delicate balancing act aimed at preventing seizures without upsetting your body chemistry or the delicate state of the fetus, you will need to prepare and proceed more carefully than most women. It's particularly important that you also do the following:

Plan Your Pregnancy!

Women usually find out that they are pregnant in the fourth to sixth week of pregnancy. By that time, the harmful effects of certain AEDs may have already occurred. Let your epileptologist know that you are planning to become pregnant as early as possible so there will be time to prepare and possibly change your medication or reduce multiple medications to a single one.

And you should follow the rules of a healthy pregnancy beginning at least three months before conception, if not earlier:

- Eat a healthful, balanced diet.

- Get plenty of sleep.

- Exercise moderately.

- Don't smoke.

- Avoid alcohol.

- Avoid caffeine.

- Keep body weight as close to ideal as possible.

Achieve Good Seizure Control Before You Conceive

Women with better seizure control before pregnancy usually have fewer seizures during pregnancy. Your epileptologist will consider changing your medication, decreasing the dosage or even stopping it, in some cases. *Do not make any medication-related decisions on your own, as the results could be disastrous.*

Consider Genetic Counseling

This can be valuable, especially if there is a history of birth defects or inherited disorders in your family. Genetic testing even in healthy individuals can help determine the risk for passing certain diseases to your baby.

Take Folic Acid and Prenatal Vitamins

It's very important that you begin taking folic acid supplements and prenatal vitamins *before* you conceive. Some AEDs may deplete the body of folic acid and deficiencies of this vitamin during early pregnancy have been linked to certain malformations. Neural tube defects (spina bifida), for example, occur just 24-28 days after conception, before most women even know they are pregnant. Unless you start taking folic acid before conception, you could easily be deficient during this critical period. It's recommend that you take 1-4 mg of folic acid plus prenatal vitamins before you start trying to conceive, and continue to take this dose throughout your pregnancy.

Consider Vitamin K

Since some AEDs may interfere with vitamin K metabolism and increase the risk of unnecessary bleeding in the baby (neonatal internal hemorrhaging), ask your obstetrician about taking 10mg vitamin K starting at 36 weeks of pregnancy as a preventive measure.

ONCE YOU'VE BECOME PREGNANT...

When you first suspect you may be pregnant, it's important that you contact your obstetrician and epileptologist immediately as you'll need to be carefully monitored. Some special concerns will include your medication and fetal testing.

Keep Taking Your Medication

Now that you're pregnant, you must continue taking your AEDs as prescribed. Do *not* alter doses or stop taking your medications without discussing your medication regimen with your doctors, as seizures during pregnancy can be life threatening for you and the baby. Blood levels of AEDs must be monitored frequently and dosages adjusted, as pregnancy alters the metabolism and may cause faster breakdown and excretion of medication, leading to breakthrough seizures.

If you do have a seizure, don't panic! Most women who have seizures during pregnancy have normal, healthy babies. But be sure to notify your epileptologist immediately and keep taking your medications as prescribed.

Consider Fetal Testing

You may want to ask your obstetrician about fetal testing that allows early detection of certain birth defects. Some of these conditions may require special attention during pregnancy. For example, some studies suggest that children with spina bifida experience a better outcome if they have surgery in utero. Other conditions, such as certain heart malformations, may require immediate surgery or a specialty team at the birth to give your baby the best chance of survival. Early diagnosis will allow your physicians to assemble that team and chose an appropriate medical facility for delivery. The tests include:

- **Maternal alpha-fetoprotein** – This blood test, performed at 15-22 weeks, indicates the likelihood that certain birth defects (such as neural tube defects) or genetic disorders are present. If the test is abnormal, further diagnostic testing may be needed to clarify the abnormality.

- **Level II ultrasound (structural)** – This detailed ultrasound is done at 16-20 weeks to assess for structural abnormalities in the fetus.

- **Amniocentesis** – This procedure, done at 15-20 weeks, involves extracting a small sample of the fluid surrounding the fetus, which is tested for indications of Down's syndrome, neural tube defects and other abnormalities.

- Even if no subsequent measures are taken, knowing in advance that such conditions exist will give you extra time to prepare for a baby with special needs.

Make a Birth Plan

A birth plan is a document that spells out the individualized care you want during labor and delivery. (To see a birth plan template, visit: http://www.womenshealthcaretopics.com/pregnancy/pregnancy_77.html.)

Designed to facilitate communication with your medical team (obstetrician and neurologist/epileptologist) during delivery, the birth plan should be shared with all parties at least one month prior to your delivery date. Then, be sure to bring it with you to the hospital for the delivery.

Before you create a birth plan, however, you should be aware of a few points: It's recommended that you give birth in a hospital; water birth is *not* recommended. And the fact that you have epilepsy is *not* a reason (by itself) for inducing labor or performing a Caesarean section.

DELIVERY

Seizures seldom occur during delivery, and most women with epilepsy are able to deliver babies without complications. But be prepared by taking the following measures:

- Inform all of your health care providers about your epilepsy and the medications you're taking.

- Always take your AEDs as prescribed throughout your entire pregnancy.

- Bring your AEDs with you to the hospital for the birth and continue to take them throughout labor and after delivery.

- Bring your birth plan with you to the hospital.

If a seizure does occur during labor, intravenous medication may be used to stop it. If the seizure is prolonged, your obstetrician may recommend a C-section delivery.

WHEN THE BABY ARRIVES...

Congratulations! Your baby has arrived and you've begun an exciting new adventure that will change your life forever. Mothers with epilepsy face the same challenges inherent in parenting a newborn that other parents face plus a couple of others. They include possible post-delivery sedation of the baby, increased blood levels of AEDs in the mother, deciding on breastfeeding while taking AEDs, and caring for an infant while being subject to seizures.

Post-Delivery Sedation of the Baby

The baby may be sedated due to exposure to AEDs in utero, particularly with Phenobarbital (Luminal®). After the medication wears off, the baby may exhibit withdrawal symptoms, although they seldom present a health risk and usually resolve quickly.

Increased Blood Levels of Medication in the Mother

During pregnancy, changes in your body may have speeded up the metabolism of your medications, requiring that you take higher dosages to prevent seizures. But during the first two months post-delivery, the process will reverse and your dosage may need to be decreased. Make sure your blood levels of AEDs are monitored regularly during this period and immediately report any side effects to your epileptologist.

Breastfeeding

Breastfeeding has significant advantages for both infant and mother, including the forging of the maternal-child bond and the transmission of antibodies, which reduces the child's risk of infection and immunological disorders. Many women also want to experience breastfeeding because they consider it an important part of being a mother. For all of these reasons, breastfeeding by mothers with epilepsy is generally recommended.

But if you're taking AEDs, you're probably concerned about passing the medication on to your baby through your breast milk. While very small amounts of *any* AED you're taking will be present in your breast milk, it will be much less than your baby was receiving in utero. It's the concentration (not just the presence) of the drug in the breast milk that is important, and this varies from medication to medication, based largely on the drug's protein binding ability.

Most drugs circulate in the mother's bloodstream bound to a protein molecule called albumin. But some circulate freely and are not protein-bound. Those that are "free" transfer into the breast milk easily, while those that are protein-bound remain in the mother's bloodstream. This means that medications with a high affinity for protein binding, like carbamazapine (Tegretol®, Carbatrol®), phenytoin (Dilantin®, Phenytek®) and valproic acid (Depakote®), will be found in breast milk in minimal amounts. But those with a low affinity for protein binding, such as ethosuximide (Zarontin®) lamotrigine (Lamictal®) and primidone (Mysoline®), may be found in breast milk in amounts large enough to affect the baby.

Other factors that determine the medication level in your baby's bloodstream include the amount of breast milk your baby drinks and how quickly he/she can eliminate the drug. If you are breastfeeding while taking AEDs, one way to minimize your baby's intake of medication is to take your dosage immediately *after* feeding the baby. This will give your body time to eliminate some of the medication before the baby feeds again.

As for the effects of AEDs in the breast milk on the baby, the most common are sedation and lethargy, which may interfere with normal growth and development. Because of this, your baby's growth and development must be carefully monitored for possible side effects, especially if you're taking:

- ethosuximide (Zarontin®)

- phenobarbital (Luminal®)

- primidone (Mysoline®)

- benzodiazepines (Valium®, Ativan®, Klonopin®)

All in all, the benefits of breastfeeding to both mother and child are believed to outweigh the risks of infant exposure to small amounts of AEDs.

Naturally, before making any decisions regarding breastfeeding while on medication, you should consult your obstetrician.

Seizure Precautions While Caring for Your Baby
Even if your seizures are under very good control, when you're caring for your baby it is wise to act as if a seizure could occur at any time. The last thing you want is to drop your child or have an accident in the bathtub because of a sudden unexpected epileptic episode.

A few simple seizure precautions can help to keep your baby safe:

- Take your medications as prescribed.

- Avoid sleep deprivation. Sleep when your baby sleeps and get somebody else to take that middle-of-the-night feeding with bottled milk! Accept all the help you can get to allow yourself time for getting the sleep you need.

- Put the baby on a blanket on the floor when you change diapers or clothing.

- Feed your baby in an infant seat on the floor.

- Use a stroller to transfer your baby from room to room, even when you're in the house.

- Fasten the safety straps whenever you put your baby in an infant seat.

- Don't give the baby a bath by yourself. When you are alone, give sponge baths on the floor.

- Avoid carrying the baby up and down stairs. Keep necessary supplies on each level of the house.

- Develop a support system of family and friends who can help you take care of the baby so you can minimize stress and get the rest you need. Hire help, if necessary!

IN A NUTSHELL

Although we've covered a lot of information in the chapter, the gist of it can be summed up in just a few sentences:

- Most women with epilepsy who become pregnant will have a healthy, uneventful pregnancy and a healthy baby. However, learning about possible risks will help you and your medical team recognize possible complications early on and treat them in a timely manner.

- Taking anti-epileptic drugs while pregnant does pose some risk to your baby, but in some cases, *not* taking them may be even more risky for your child. (See your doctor to find out what's right for you.)

- By planning your pregnancy, you can start taking prenatal vitamins/folic acid and get your medications adjusted *before* you conceive, making a good pregnancy outcome much more likely.

- Finally, establishing a trusting relationship with the members of your medical team prior to pregnancy, and maintaining good communication with them throughout should help you get through your pregnancy with a minimum of trouble.

CHAPTER TWELVE
PRACTICAL ISSUES

Thirty-nine year-old Jessie has had epilepsy since she was a small child. Although it is usually fairly well-controlled, she does experience a breakthrough seizure from time to time. But Jessie never really thought of herself as "disabled" until two years ago, when she and her husband got divorced and she lost custody of her son. Now Jessie declares, "The courts, my ex-husband and even my own parents decided I was unfit to care for my son because of my seizures. If that's not disabled and unfair, I don't know what is."

Is epilepsy a disability? Setting aside the legal issues, I tell my patients to beware of adopting a belief that becomes a self-fulfilling prophecy, as in, "I have a disabling disorder; I am disabled; I can't do things; why try?" Once you start thinking of yourself as "disabled," your epilepsy will become a disability and will begin to define your life, who you are and what you can do. Your life will become centered around "I can't."

I urge you always to strive to do the opposite. Live life to the fullest by focusing on all of the things you *can* do (and there are a lot of them). Take control of your life, become an active part of your treatment team, and embrace life! This way of thinking will energize and empower you.

Michael began experiencing partial-onset seizures at the age of 5. At age 20, he got a job working in an assembly plant. "I told them straight out when I was interviewed that I have seizures," Michael said. "They asked me what that meant; then they asked me if I thought I could do the job. I said 'yes,' and they agreed to try me out. I've been working at the plant for almost twenty years now! I really like working there and hanging out with the guys. I feel like I belong."

A few years ago, Michael had surgery to remove the seizure focus in his brain, and that made his good life even better. As he tells, it, "Before my surgery, when I still had seizures, the people at work just made sure I wasn't around any dangerous machinery and was never alone in the plant. But there was still a lot of stuff I could do to be useful. And since my surgery, I got a really important job promotion. Now I enjoy working even more and feel really proud of myself."

Like Michael, you can grab hold of your life and take control. Find ways to work around the obstacles in your life and keep a positive outlook – there are solutions!

But in order to truly regain control, you must learn to handle certain practical issues related to epilepsy, including seizure-related emergencies, transportation, safety, traveling, exercising and playing sports.

SEIZURE-RELATED CRITICAL SITUATIONS

Because seizures produce uncontrolled physical activity, there is a real risk of injury, especially if you are engaged in any activity that requires full awareness (driving, operating power tools, swimming, climbing ladders and so on). Ask your doctor which activities are considered to be safe. And be aware that even something as simple as walking through your house while holding a lit candle can be dangerous if a seizure occurs.

Most seizures don't require emergency care unless you get injured. However, there are two seizure-related conditions that automatically fall into the critical category – *status epilepticus* and *sudden unexplained death due to epilepsy.*

Status Epilepticus

The term "status epilepticus" refers to any uninterrupted seizure that lasts longer than five minutes. When a seizure lasts this long, it is unlikely to stop spontaneously and will require immediate medical intervention. Tell your family, friends, caregivers and workmates that if you have a seizure that lasts longer than two to three minutes, they should call 911 immediately.

Status epilepticus is typically brought on by the sudden cessation of seizure medication, alcohol withdrawal, brain infections such as meningitis or encephalitis, stroke or traumatic brain injury. A serious condition that takes 50,000 American lives each year, status epilepticus can take several different forms, including:

- **Partial motor status epilepticus** – This prolonged seizure involves just one part of the brain. The person is awake and talking/interacting normally, but has persistent rhythmic jerking on one side of the body, say the hand, arm or face. It requires emergency treatment, but is not usually as life-threatening as other forms.

- **Generalized convulsive status epilepticus** - This prolonged seizure involves the entire brain, and produces convulsive activity in all four extremities coupled with a lack of responsiveness. This life-threatening condition requires urgent medical evaluation and treatment.

- **Nonconvulsive status epilepticus** – This seizure, which could involve part of the brain or the entire organ, is far less dramatic than generalized convulsive status epilepticus, and produces subtle symptoms such as blinking, staring or confusion – or no obvious signs at all. It is less dangerous than the generalized convulsive type, but still requires prompt recognition and treatment. A continuous EEG recording is the only way to diagnose non-convulsive status epilepticus.

- **Myoclonic status epilepticus** - Another seizure that involves the entire brain, this form produces prolonged jerking that could involve all four extremities and be associated with lack of responsiveness. It is usually caused by a profound lack of oxygen to the brain due to heart dysfunction, but may also occur in those with myoclonic epilepsy.

Prognosis depends on the cause and duration of the status epilepticus. In general, if the condition is the result of injury due to a lack of oxygen to the brain, as in a stroke or heart dysfunction, the outcome will be less favorable because of the possibility of irreversible brain injury. Obviously, the sooner status epilepticus is recognized and treated, the better the outcome.

Sudden Unexplained Death in Epilepsy

Sudden, unexpected death in a person with epilepsy (SUDEP) is a genuine bolt out of the blue as it can strike a person who is otherwise in good health. There may be no obvious cause of death because no one witnessed the seizure and the victim didn't drown or suffer any seizure-related trauma. Suspected causes of SUDEP are airway obstruction during or after a seizure, apnea (pauses in breathing), pulmonary edema (lungs filled with fluid) and irregular heartbeat. Genetics may also play a role.

Approximately 1 out of 1,000 people with epilepsy falls victim to SUDEP, which usually strikes those between 25-50 years of age who have severe epilepsy. The highest risk of SUDEP is seen in those who have had epilepsy longer than two years, have poor seizure control, and experience generalized tonic-clonic seizures. Other risk factors include profound intellectual disabilities, seizures during sleep, and taking more than two prescribed seizure medications (which is probably related to poor seizure control). Some who succumb to SUDEP are found to have low blood levels of seizure medication, indicating they were not taking the full dosage of prescribed medicine.

Because we don't yet know what causes SUDEP, it's hard to say how to prevent it. However, it is a very good idea to take your seizure medications exactly as prescribed and get your medication levels monitored regularly through blood tests, when indicated by your doctor. Also, be sure to fill your prescriptions regularly so you don't run out of medication and go to all of your follow-up appointments. Although recent research is suggesting that some cases of SUDEP may be associated to genetic mutations that cause a potentially deadly electrical disorder of the heart, genetic testing is not yet a standard recommendation. Certainly, consider getting a second opinion at an epilepsy center if your seizures remain frequent and uncontrolled even though you are faithfully following your treatment plan.

On a brighter note, people with mild epilepsy appear to be at minimal risk of SUDEP, and SUDEP doesn't seem to affect those who have outgrown childhood epilepsy.

THE SEIZURE PREPAREDNESS PLAN

While I urge my patients to expect the best, it's necessary to prepare for the possibility of future seizures by developing a Seizure Preparedness Plan. The plan, which is for your friends, family, caregivers, or anyone else who may be with you when a seizure strikes, should include the following directives (or something similar):

In Case of Seizure:

- Please keep calm and stay with me until the seizure ends.

- These symptoms/behaviors will tell you that I'm having a seizure: (list specific characteristics of your seizures, for example, falling, jerking limbs, etc.) _____

- The things you should do to ensure my safety are: (for example, gently move me away from danger, if possible; loosen any restrictive clothing, etc.) _____
  _____

- Please *do not* put anything in my mouth during the seizure!

- Please observe me carefully so you can describe everything you saw during the seizure. I'll report what you've said to my doctor and it may help with my treatment.

- Look at the time when the seizure starts. Please call 911 if the seizure is prolonged (lasts longer than two to three minutes), is associated with breathing difficulties, causes injury, or becomes a series of seizures. Brief seizures that end spontaneously without injury do not require a 911 call, but may require a call to my doctor. My doctor's phone number is:
  _____

- If several seizures occur in a row, please give me my rescue seizure medication as follows: (list instructions obtained from your doctor. If you wear a VNS, include instructions to swipe it once over the implant.)
  _____
  _____

- After the seizure, please help me find a place to rest. It is also important that I get regular meals and take my seizure medications on schedule.

If you have a school-age child with epilepsy, the Seizure Preparedness Plan should be given to the school nurse or other appropriate school official, as well as the teachers, coaches, camp director, camp counselor, babysitters and anyone else who may be caring for the child. Some parents shy away from sharing information about their child's epilepsy with school to avoid stigmatization. But I urge them to consider how important it is for key personnel to be prepared in the event of an emergency.

DRIVING

Marcia, a 40 year-old executive assistant, hasn't been able to drive for the past 23 years due to epileptic seizures caused by a brain tumor. She is still furious about it, saying, "Can you believe that I only got to drive one year of my life? As soon as I got my license, my dad bought me a brand new Toyota Corolla and I felt all grown up and independent. Then, out of the blue, I had a seizure, was diagnosed with a brain tumor, and kept having seizures even after the tumor was removed. So now here I am, still not driving at age 40! And unless I get these seizures under control, I'll never get my driver's license back."

Losing the ability to drive because of continuing seizures can create a loss of independence and feeling of isolation that is nothing short of devastating. And while the suspension of driving privileges makes life more difficult, especially if you live in an area that doesn't have excellent public/alternative transportation, it's important to remember that these laws protect the safety of *everyone* on the road.

However, the laws do vary from state to state. For example, some states require the doctor to report a patient with seizures to the appropriate state department, while other expect the patient to divulge their seizure activity. Some states will reinstate a driver's license after a person has been seizure-free for as little as three months. (See Appendix 2: Seizure-Related Driving Regulations – Listed by State to find your state's requirements.) Certain rules and regulations will apply to specific kinds of licenses, depending on whether it's a regular driver's license, a commercial license or other kind of license. The good news is there is a real chance that you'll be able to drive again in the future.

For more information, see http://www.fmcsa.dot.gov/documents/ neuro2.pdf

What About Your I.D.?

Just because you don't have a driver's license doesn't mean you won't have a legal form of identification. Your state's Department of Motor Vehicles can issue a Photo Identification Card to use for I.D. when you make purchases, board an airplane or do anything that requires identification. Some states now offer on-line applications to make the process easier.

Until you can regain your driving privileges, the best way to take back control of your life is to use alternate means of getting around. Look into public transportation, taxis and paratransit systems in your area. Community organizations, Medicaid, Veteran's aid and family and friends are other viable options.

Public Transportation

If you live in a metropolitan area, you might have access to an extensive, easy-to-use public transportation system. And many times people with a disability can get a reduced-fare card. Check with your local transportation authority for details and applications.

Taxis

Taxis are generally available in all areas, including the very rural. If you are going to schedule regular trips, look for a cab company that will offer you a reduced fare in exchange for booking with them exclusively.

Paratransit Systems

These public transportation systems are designed for people with disabilities who are unable to use standard buses or trains. Run by local or state governments, non-profit agencies, or private transportation companies, they typically charge a reduced or nominal per-trip fee, or may even offer free rides.

Check out the following websites to find out if you qualify for paratransit transportation and to locate a paratransit system in your state:

- **Americans with Disabilities Act (ADA) Paratransit Eligibility Manual**
  http://ntl.bts.gov/DOCS/ada.html.

- **Disability.gov**
  http://www.disability.gov/transportation. (Find the red bar at the lower left marked "Information by State" and enter your state in the box directly beneath it.)

Community Organizations

Your local religious organizations and civic groups may link you to volunteers who can help you get around. While they probably won't be able to take you to and from work on a daily basis, the volunteers may be happy to drive you to a medical appointment, the supermarket or a monthly support group.

Medicaid Assistance

Transportation benefits for Medicaid recipients vary from state to state. Travel expenses to and from medical appointments or to pick up prescriptions are covered by most plans. Some plans also offer reimbursement for transportation to events like support groups. Ask your Medicaid service coordinator about the options available in your state. (See Appendix 1: Resources.)

Veterans Aid

Many programs help veterans with their transportation needs. Check with your local Department of Veterans Affairs or visit:

- **National Resource Web Directory of National Public Transportation Services Available for Veterans**: http://www.nationalresourcedirectory.gov/transportation_ and_travel; then click on "Transportation Assistance and Public Transportation"

- **The Disabled American Veterans Transportation Network** http://www.dav.org/volunteers/Ride.aspx

Family and Friends

No one wants to burden loved ones with continual requests for rides, but keep in mind that many people really do like to feel useful. Family members and close friends might welcome the opportunity to help you when other options have been exhausted. Just ask. Offer to reimburse them for gas and let them drive your car, if you have one. The bonus can be extra time spent with a great person!

SAFETY IN AND OUT OF THE HOME

If you're like most people with epilepsy, you live at home, rather than in a nursing facility. And it's quite possible that you are alone there for lengthy periods of time. Thus, it's important to make your home as safe as possible in case you have a seizure when there's no one around to help you.

Safety at Home

Make your home as safe as possible by doing the following:

- Make sure that your floors are carpeted and any sharp corners (e.g., table corners) are padded to reduce the risk of injury due to a fall.

- Don't smoke.

- Don't light a fire or a candle when you are home alone.

- Make sure the drains in your bathtub and shower are working properly to prevent drowning should you lose consciousness while showering.

- Set your water temperature to a moderate level to avoid being scalded if you lose consciousness while running the hot water.

- Don't take a bath in deep water, to prevent drowning.

- Don't lock the bathroom door (you can use a sign on the outside to indicate it is occupied). Install a bathroom door that opens outward for easier access, in case you have a seizure and fall against the door.

- Use plastic glasses and dinnerware instead of glass and china to keep from cutting yourself if you lose consciousness while holding them.

- Keep your smoke detector active.

- Avoid cooking on a stove and opt in favor of using the microwave.

- Place window guards, if appropriate.

Some people also use medical alert systems that notify emergency personnel that they've fallen and need assistance. Baby monitors can be helpful to parents of babies or young children who have epileptic seizures during sleep, as they can pick up unusual sounds.

I'm often asked about epilepsy detectors, which are devices that monitor movement, breathing, and/or detect urine or vomit in the bed and send warning signals if something is amiss. While it's an intriguing idea, none of them are FDA-approved for home use.

You'll find more extensive home safety recommendations at:

- **Epilepsy Foundation – Home Safety**
  http://www.epilepsyfoundation.org

Safety Away From Home

There are also several ways to ensure your safety when you leave your home. For example:

- Always tell your family and/or friends where you are going and when you expect to return.

- Don't leave home without your cell phone (if you cannot afford one, many states will now provide persons who qualify with one with a limited number of minutes).

- Wear a Medic-Alert bracelet and/or jewelry printed with your medical information.

- Carry an index card with you with any important information first responders would need to know about your seizures, treatment, doctor's contact numbers, and so forth

- Put your emergency contact numbers on speed-dial on your cell phone and have them in your address book under "In case of emergency" (ICE).

- Don't drive without medical permission.

- Keep a supply of rescue medication on hand.

- Stay away from the tracks at train and subway stations.

- If you fall frequently during seizures, consider taking an elevator instead of an escalator or stairs.

TRAVELING

Traveling out of town can require more extensive preparations, but don't let this stop you from getting out there and living your life! Do discuss your plans with your doctor in advance, and if you have frequent seizures or become confused during seizures, don't travel alone.

General Travel Guidelines
- Give your friends and family a copy of your travel itinerary, with phone numbers and addresses where you can be reached.

- Become familiar with the hospitals in the areas you are visiting, in case of emergency.

- Bring an adequate supply of seizure medication with you.

- If the trip is a long one, consider finding a medical provider in the area to provide refills. However, be aware that not all countries have access to every seizure medication prescribed in the United States. Find out in advance which ones are available, and talk to your doctor about other medicines that are acceptable.

- Longer flights and jet lag can cause disrupted sleep, which can trigger a seizure. Talk to your doctor about getting a prescription sleep aid for the trip.

- Avoid excessive alcohol.

- Eat regular meals.

- Don't forget to consider time zone changes when taking your medications. Take the medication as close as possible to the time you would be taking it at home.

- If you travelling to a foreign country, consider learning basic phrases to request medical assistance such as "I need help" and "Where is the hospital?" Carry an index card with all your most important health information in the country's language.

- Prepare a plan for an emergency trip back home. Discuss this plan with someone you trust before you go.

- Consider buying traveler's insurance to cover overseas medical costs if needed or the premature cancelation of your trip.

- Consult your epilpetologist about any vaccinations you may be receiving as they could potentially interact with your regular medications.

- Airport security only allows us to carry liquids up to 100 ml. Contact the airline and get a letter from your doctor to allow you to board with all the medication you may need. Do not put your medications in your suitcase. A lost suitcase could derail your trip terribly.

Traveling Alone

Obviously, it's never a good idea to travel alone if you have active seizures, but sometimes it may be necessary. If you do travel alone, be sure to:

- Wear a Medic-Alert bracelet/necklace that includes a description of your seizure(s).

- Carry a list on your person of all of your current medications (plus enough medicine to last you from start to end of your trip).

- Carry emergency contact information on your person, either on an index card or numbers programmed into your cell phone and listed under contacts as ICE (In Case of Emergency).

- Disclose your seizure history to transportation personnel and provide them with a letter from your doctor.

- Let the flight attendants, conductor or driver know that you have epilepsy.

- If you have a VNS device implanted, carry a VNS registration card so that people will know that you cannot get an MRI, should not have deep heat treatment and so on.

To learn more about traveling with epilepsy, see:

- **Air Travel Guidelines**
  http://www.epilepsyfoundation.org
-
- **Epilepsy Foundation - Transportation Guide**
  http://www.epilepsyfoundation.org

EXERCISE AND SPORTS

People with epilepsy sometimes worry that exercise might trigger a seizure, but this is very rare. For the vast majority of those with epilepsy, the benefits of exercise far outweigh the risks. Regular exercise helps reduce anxiety and depression, boost energy, promote better sleep, improve the sex life, combat chronic disease, lessen social isolation, and improve overall health – all of which are important to good physical and psychological health. Recreational activities can contribute a great deal to a person's overall happiness and greatly improve the social life. But even more to the point, there is some evidence that exercise may actually help reduce both the susceptibility to seizures and seizure frequency, possibly through its role in stress reduction.[2] (Stress is an important trigger of epileptic seizures.)

Now this doesn't mean that *all* types of exercise are necessarily good for those with epilepsy. It will depend very much on the individual and the type/severity/frequency of the seizures. In general, let common sense be your guide when deciding which activities need special gear (such as a helmet) and which must be avoided completely. And always check with your doctor *before* engaging in any kind of athletic activity. Basic rules of thumb: keep yourself hydrated, avoid overexertion, take breaks when needed, follow safety guidelines.

Most people with epilepsy can safely participate in most sports, even when their seizures are not fully controlled. This means that just taking a few extra safety precautions may be enough to get you into the game! For a general idea about the precautions that should be taken when engaging in various sports, see the following table.

Note: Some activities require full concentration, and any loss of consciousness may lead to injury and/or death. You should discuss with your doctor which activities are appropriate for you

---

[2] Arida RM, Scorza FA, Terra VC, et al. Physical exercise in epilepsy: what kind of stressor is it? *Epilepsy Behav* 2009;16(3):381-87.

Table 1: *SAFETY PRECAUTIONS WHEN ENGAGING IN SPORTS*

ACTIVITY	PRECAUTIONS
ATVs	• Your state or country may not require a driver's license but it is a high risk activity and should be avoided
Baseball	• Wear protective clothing: ✓elbow or knee pads ✓helmet ✓protective eyeglasses or goggles Let your coach know
Basketball	• Wear protective clothing: ✓elbow or knee pads ✓consider a helmet ✓protective eyeglasses or goggles Let your coach know
Bike Riding	• Avoid busy streets • Ride on bike paths • Ride on side streets • Wear a helmet and reflective clothing If possible ride with a buddy
Boxing	• High risk activity - should be avoided by all
Bungee Jumping	• High risk activity - should be avoided by all
Canoeing/ Kayaking	• Never canoe/kayak alone; take a "buddy" who knows seizure first aid. • Always wear a high quality, well-fitting life vest when near the water to prevent drowning and a helmet if needed. • Avoid closed kayaks to avoid being trapped underwater if it flips over

Football	• Wear protective clothing: ✓ elbow or knee pads ✓ helmet ✓ protective eyeglasses or goggles Let your coach know
Gymnastics	• Have a "buddy" when using equipment like balance beams, parallel bars or when vaulting • Consider a helmet when using a balance beam or parallel bars or when vaulting • Use a shock-absorbing mat • **Let your coach know**
***Hang Gliding**	• High risk activity - should be avoided by individuals with uncontrolled seizures Tandem hang gliding with an experienced instructor may be a possibility (discuss this over with your doctor and the instructor)
Horseback Riding	• Wear protective clothing: ✓ elbow,knee pads and perhaps an inflatable vest ✓ helmet (titanium is preferred) ✓ protective eyeglasses or goggles Ride within your mastery level
Ice Hockey	• Wear protective clothing: ✓ elbow or knee pads ✓ helmet ✓ protective eyeglasses or goggles Let your coach know
Jet Skiing	• High risk activity - should be avoided by individuals with uncontrolled seizures
Jogging	• Only in safe surroundings (preferably on a track) ✓ safety gear ✓ consider being with a buddy

Martial Arts: Karate, Tai Kwando, Judo	• Wear Protective gear including a helmet Work on shock-absorbing mats Let your teacher know so that blows to the head are avoided during practice.
*Mountain Climbing	• High risk activity - should be avoided by individuals with uncontrolled seizures
Pilates	• Have a 'buddy" when using equipment • Working on the mat rather than on the machines might be preferable for some
*Rappelling	• High risk activity - should be avoided by individuals with uncontrolled seizures
*Rock Climbing	• High risk activity - should be avoided by individuals with uncontrolled seizures
Rollerblading	• Wear protective clothing: ✓ elbow or knee pads ✓ helmet ✓ protective eyeglasses or goggles Have a buddy when possible Avoid busy streets
Rugby	• Wear protective clothing: ✓ elbow or knee pads ✓ helmet ✓ protective eyeglasses or goggles Let your coach know
*Scuba Diving	• High risk activity - should be avoided by individual with uncontrolled seizures However, depending on what country you are in, local laws may allow you to scuba dive after a certain number of years of seizure freedom and being off medications.

Skateboarding	• Wear protective clothing: ✓ elbow or knee pads ✓ helmet ✓ protective eyeglasses or goggles Avoid busy streets Consider skateboarding with a buddy
Skiing	• Dress for warmth • Wear protective gear including a helmet • Consider a safety strap when riding the t-bar or a modified climbing harness • Have a "buddy" • Don't go off open trails Ski within your mastery level
Snorkeling	• High risk activity - should be avoided by individuals with uncontrolled seizures
***Skydiving**	• High risk activity - should be avoided by individuals with uncontrolled seizures An option may be to tandem sky-dive with an instructor. Each case is different and you would need to discuss this option thoroughly with your doctor and the instructor
Soccer	• Wear protective clothing: ✓ elbow or knee pads ✓ helmet ✓ protective eyeglasses or goggles Let your coach know
Surfing/Wind Surfing	• High risk activity - should be avoided by individuals with uncontrolled seizures

Swimming	• Never swim alone. Have a "buddy" who knows seizure first aid • Always wear a high-quality, well-fitting life vest when near the water to help prevent drowning. • Inform the lifeguard about your condition if swimming in a pool (explain what your seizures look like) Avoid swimming in open water.
Tai chi	• Consider a shock-absorbing mat
Weight lifting	• Work with a buddy who is attentive and aware of your condition ✓ shock absorbing mat ✓ avoid placing yourself underneath weights or in other dangerous positions
Working out at the gym	• On the treadmill: attach yourself to the auto-stop cord ✓ take frequent breaks ✓ keep yourself hydrated ✓ avoid over-exertion ✓ work out on a shock absorbing mat
Yoga	• Consider a shock-absorbing mat= Avoid some of the more intense yoga variants that involve high temperatures or extreme breathing

Always wear a Medic-Alert bracelet or necklace and carry your medical information when engaging in sports. You should also enter your emergency contact information in your cell phone under ICE (In Case of Emergency). Decide who most needs to know about your epilepsy to assure your safety. This could be a coach, trainer, life guard, team members, etc.

SOCIAL ACTIVITIES AND RELATIONSHIPS

If your seizures are uncontrolled, it can be difficult to participate in social events, visit with friends and enjoy leisure activities. You can easily become isolated because you are afraid of having a seizure in public, you fear rejection if people find out about your condition, you may be unable to drive or go places by yourself, and/or your activities may be restricted due to safety concerns. There may also be financial restrictions due to unemployment or underemployment. And if you've been isolated for a long time, you may feel awkward in social settings just because you're not used to being "in the swing of things."

Obviously, achieving good seizure control is of utmost importance in the regaining of your social confidence. But some people still shy away from socializing even when their seizures are unlikely to occur. I want to remind everyone who feels that epilepsy is a reason to stay away from others that *epilepsy does not define you; it is something you have and that you can learn to live with*. When you come to see epilepsy as a life challenge, not a life sentence, you will find the courage to move forward in life and make yourself the person you want to be and who you'll be happy to be.

In the meantime, I urge you to step out of your comfort zone and push yourself to engage in life. Take a chance and initiate some new friendships. Some may not take, but those that do will increase your confidence, social sphere and enjoyment of life. Pursue a career, big or small; it will broaden your life and make you feel productive. Participate in your community, as the best way to feel good about yourself is to help others. And be aware that eliminating the stigma of epilepsy is your responsibility, too. Explain the disorder to anyone who will listen.

CHAPTER THIRTEEN
EPILEPSY AND THE WORK PLACE

Work, an important and often central part of life for adults, goes beyond simply earning a living. Most of us identify ourselves in terms of what we do: carpenter, nurse, bus driver, teacher, programmer, attorney, hairdresser, and so on. If you're not working due to seizures, or if your present job is limited for that reason, you may feel you lack an identity or are "less than." While there's no doubt that seizures can be a hindrance, they don't have to be career-killers. In fact, the odds are very good that even with epilepsy, you can still work successfully in your chosen field.

In this chapter, we will look at some important issues concerning epilepsy and work/careers, from choosing a career path, to fighting against discrimination on the job.

CHOOSING A CAREER

If you have never worked or only worked sporadically, your first step should be to select a career path, a *realistic* choice based on your abilities, experience, transportation limitations, and other factors. Unless you have a burning desire to go into a certain field, you might find it helpful to seek professional assistance in selecting your career.

If you're in school, visit the counseling department for career guidance. If you are not in school, be aware that every state has a

Vocational Rehabilitation Department or a similar program that offers aptitude tests to help you select the occupation that best suits you, and other forms of job assistance. To locate an office close to you, visit: http://www.disability.gov/employment, then search for your state's Vocational Rehabilitation Services Department.

Here are a few more helpful websites:

- **Assessment & Career Exploration**
  https://www.disability.gov/employment/career_planning

- **Bureau of Labor Statistics: Career Guide to Industries**
  http://www.bls.gov/oco/cg/home.htm

- **Workforce Investment Act Training Programs**
  http://www.careeronestop.org/WiaProviderSearch.asp

- **Epilepsy Life Links – Epilepsy Support - Employment**
  http://www.epilepsylifelinks.com/services_employment.php

Also many states have a job tab on their official website where job fairs are announced and job postings can be found.

LANDING THAT JOB

Once you've selected your career path, it's time to start a job search. In addition to the standard means of finding a job, consider visiting a One-Stop Career Center in your area. These centers offer job listings and career counseling and can walk you through the job search process – from locating an attractive position to helping you with the job application. For a link to One-Stop Career Centers, visit:

- **The U.S. Department of Labor**
  http://www.dol.gov/dol/topic/training/onestop.htm

Another helpful site for career planning is Disability.gov, which has links to many sites that can assist in your job search:

- **Disability. Gov**
  https://www.disability.gov/employment/career_planning

Writing a Great Resume

Once you have identified some possible job openings, you'll need to let your prospective employers know that you're that special person they're looking for – and that generally requires writing a great resume. If you're like many people, you may dread resume writing. But think of it as your opportunity to shine! Presenting a high quality resume and cover letter will go a long way toward getting you that all-important first interview, so spend some time on it. Your vocational counselor will assist you, but it's also important that you understand how to do it yourself.

Start by gathering information about all of your previous jobs, volunteer activities, education, sports and anything else that might be even slightly relevant. It's best to have too much material to work with! But don't let a short work history discourage you. Even if you haven't held a paying position before, think about your life experiences that will demonstrate your abilities. Did you ever babysit, mow lawns, shovel snow, or volunteer at your church or school or in the community? Even these seemingly unrelated tasks can help you build an appealing resume that showcases your abilities. Come prepared to meet your vocational counselor with a list of your past activities, and don't forget to include hobbies, clubs and associations.

You can find information about resumes, strategies for writing good resumes and more at:

- **Career One Stop: Pathways to Career Success**
  http://www.careeronestop.org/ResumeGuide/
  MoreSampleResumes.aspx

What to Disclose About Your Epilepsy

You may be wondering when, if ever, you should tell a prospective employer that you have epilepsy. The answer is there is no "right" moment to offer this information. You must decide for yourself whether to tell a prospective or actual employer about your epilepsy and, if so, when to do so. You may decide not to disclose this information during the job interview unless you are asked one of the very few allowed questions. In most cases, prospective employers can ask only if you have any limitations that would prevent you from performing the job in question. They cannot request information about specific diseases, medications, hospitalizations and so on. The U.S. Equal Employment Opportunity Commission puts it this way: "Before making an offer of employment, an employer may not ask job applicants about the existence, nature, or severity of a disability. Applicants may be asked about their ability to perform job functions."

Once you're offered a job, however, the employer can probe for more information. According to the Equal Employment Opportunity Commission, "A job offer may be conditioned on the results of a medical examination, but only if the examination is required for all entering employees in the same job category. Medical examinations of employees must be job-related and consistent with business necessity."

The Epilepsy Foundation has prepared a helpful chart examining the pros and cons of disclosing your epilepsy at various points, from the time you fill out a job application until after you're on the job. For more information, visit:

- **Epilepsy Foundation: Pros & Cons of Disclosing Epilepsy**
  http://www.epilepsyfoundation.org/livingwithepilepsy/employmenttopics/disclosing.cfm

IF TROUBLE STRIKES AT WORK

Let's imagine that you have landed a job and everything seems to be going well. Then one day you suddenly have a seizure at work. Everyone is very concerned and helpful, but the following week you are terminated. You've never had a bad review and there are no warnings in your personnel file. Is this discrimination or a coincidence?

Or imagine that you normally work the morning shift at a large manufacturing plant and one day your boss tells you that you'll have to rotate between the morning and late afternoon shifts. This would be disastrous for you because your seizures tend to occur in the evening. Also, the constant change in shifts would certainly interfere with your sleep, raising your overall risk of seizures. You explain that you have epilepsy and would like to remain on the morning shift, but your boss is not sympathetic. "You're doing the rotating shifts or you're fired," he says. Are these your only two choices?

These and other work situations may be covered by the Americans with Disabilities Act (ADA), a federal law that offers protection to those with disabilities who work for companies with 15 or more employees. Most states have their own laws supplementing the ADA, and they sometimes apply to smaller companies as well. Depending on the size of your company, your job-related duties, and certain other factors, you may find that you have a great deal of legal protection.

The ADA protects against discrimination in all employment practices, including job application procedures, hiring, firing, training, pay, promotions, benefits and leave. You also have a right to be free from harassment because of your disability, and an employer may not fire or discipline you for asserting your rights under the ADA. Most importantly, you have a right to request a reasonable accommodation for the hiring process and on the job.

A reasonable accommodation is any change or adjustment in a job, the work environment or the way things are usually done that would allow you to apply for that job, perform essential job functions, or enjoy equal access to benefits available to other individuals in the workplace. Some of the most common types of accommodations include:

- Time off for treatment of the disability (i.e. Doctor appointments)

- Physical changes, such as a ramp into a building or a special computer screen

- Breaks scheduled around your need to take medications

One example of a reasonable accommodation is changing the lighting around your work station if the current lighting might trigger a seizure. Another is giving you time off to try a new medication if your request is supported by a doctor's note.

If you think you might need an accommodation when applying for or performing a job, let the employer know that you need an adjustment or change because of your disability. You do not need to complete any special forms or use technical language. Once you have made the request, your employer should discuss the available options with you. Bear in mind, however, that it's possible for people to disagree about what is reasonable, so some back-and-forth may be required even with fair-minded employers. And realize that you must be able to perform the essential functions of your job with the accommodation. If you cannot perform the essential functions, even when the accommodation has been provided, your employer can justifiably terminate you.

Some employers may try to find a comparable position for you. For example, if driving is an important part of your job and you can no longer do so even with a reasonable accommodation, the employer may offer you a comparable position that does not require driving. But this is not required, especially if the employer can prove that offering a comparable position creates undue hardship.

If you feel that you are being discriminated against because of your epilepsy, there is help. First, you might want to discuss your concerns with people you trust, like your family, close friends or members of your treatment team. They may be able to help you decide if it's truly discrimination or you might be misinterpreting an action or a behavior. If you still feel that the possibility of discrimination is real, contact the Equal Employment Opportunity Commission (EEOC). They will help you decide if you should file a charge of discrimination. There are strict time frames for filing charges of employment discrimination, so be sure to file as soon as possible once you believe discrimination has taken place. For more information, visit:

- **Equal Employment Opportunity Commission – Disability Discrimination**
  http://www.eeoc.gov/laws/types/disability.cfm

Other helpful websites:

- **Americans with Disabilities Act: Guide to Disabilities Rights Laws**
  http://www.ada.gov/cguide.htm

  Fact Sheet: Questions and Answers About Epilepsy In the Workplace
  http://www.eeoc.gov/facts/epilepsy.html

- **Jeanne A. Carpenter Epilepsy Legal Defense Fund**
  http://www.epilepsyfoundation.org/epilepsylegal

MILITARY SERVICE AND EPILEPSY

Many young men and women consider it an honor and a privilege to serve in the military. And along with the honor and privilege come the benefits of travel, intrigue, and a well-earned college education. A military career can offer an adventurous short-term job or a lifelong career. But is it possible to serve if you have epilepsy?

The armed forces are not required to follow the same non-discrimination laws that guide the non-military workforce. There is a concern that those diagnosed with epilepsy may pose a risk to themselves as well as their fellow soldiers. (Having a seizure during battle or in some other hazardous situation could lead to disastrous results.) However, this does not mean that a military career is out of the question.

Currently, applicants to most branches of the military are considered if there has been no seizure activity since the age of five, or the applicant has been seizure-free without medication for five years immediately prior to application. The standard for flight training in the Air Force is more rigorous: anyone who has a history of a convulsive disorder is barred. The only exception is an applicant with seizures that were related to a febrile illness that occurred before the age of five. These applicants may be accepted if the electroencephalogram (EEG) is normal.

Do I Need to Disclose My Epilepsy When Applying for Military Service?

The application for military service does include questions about medical conditions. (Remember, certain anti-discrimination laws do *not* apply in the military.) Being less than truthful on your military application constitutes falsifying a legal document, an action that carries severe legal penalties. So it is important that you honestly answer all questions, including those related to your medical history.

What Happens If I Have a Seizure After I Enlist?

Immediate discharge of a person who develops epilepsy while enlisted is no longer required, but it is quite likely. The armed forces separation regulations are very clear concerning convulsive disorders, and state that : "...when seizures are not adequately controlled (complete freedom from seizures of any type) by standard drugs which are relatively nontoxic and which do not require frequent clinical and laboratory re-evaluation," the person will be evaluated by the Medical Review Board of that particular military branch.

The Board will then make recommendations about retention, possible reassignment, or dismissal. If you are dismissed, be sure that your records indicate that you received a medical discharge, and that all of the information in your service record is accurate. Otherwise, you may not receive optimal benefits and credit for your service.

For additional information visit:

- **Epilepsy Foundation: Military Service**
  http://www.epilepsyfoundation.org/livingwiththepilepsy/employmenttopics/safetysensitivejobs/militaryservice.cfm

  Epilepsy Foundation: Veterans: What You Need to Know: http://www.epilepsyfoundation.org/resources/veterans.cfm

- **Epilepsy Life Links Veterans Programs**
  http://www.epilepsylifelinks.com/services_veterans.php

Remember: Epilepsy is *not* your identity and should never be seen as a reason that you cannot work and get ahead in life. It is something that you have – just as other people have diabetes, high blood pressure or a particular psychological condition – but it is *never* who you are. Many people with epilepsy work steadily and have successful careers. You, too, can join their ranks!

CHAPTER FOURTEEN
LEGAL ISSUES

————————————————— ● —————————————————

The Americans with Disabilities Act (ADA) and other laws provide protection against discrimination at work, but what about when you're out with friends, walking down the street or applying for insurance? Or suppose you find yourself in financial need? Can you get help? You have rights that you may not be aware of, and forms of assistance are available that can help you through these rough spots. Let's take a look at certain hypothetical situations so you can find out what your rights are and how the law protects you.

ASKED TO LEAVE POST-SEIZURE

Let's say you're standing in the lobby of a movie theatre waiting to buy some popcorn and you have a seizure. Fortunately, you're with a companion who helps you recover quickly, get into the theatre and settle into your seat. But before the show begins, the theatre manager approaches you and asks you to leave, citing the fear that you may have another seizure and injure yourself in their facility. He gives you enough money to cover the cost of your ticket and refreshments and escorts you to the door. Must you leave?

The answer is no. Federal law states that it is unlawful for a public facility to disqualify you from participating in an event or enjoying the same activities as everyone else because of your epilepsy. It is *not* necessary to refrain from engaging in activities you enjoy, or allow others to keep you away. And it's not good for you, either; it can lead to depression, isolation, a lack of physical fitness and the downgrading of your health in general.

The best way to fight back is to know your rights and speak up! It's important that you keep epilepsy "in its place" and not allow anyone or anything to prevent you from participating in reasonable social and recreational activities. To learn about the laws that protect people with epilepsy or other disabilities, see the following websites:

- **Americans with Disabilities Act – Title III** http://www.ada.gov/reg3a.html
- **Epilepsy Foundation: Discrimination by Public Accommodations** http://www.epilepsyfoundation. org/resources/epilepsy/loader.cfm?csModule=security/ getfile&PageID=21494)

- **Section 504 of the Rehabilitation Act of 1973** http://www. hhs.gov/ocr/civilrights/resources/factsheets/504.pdf

ARRESTED DUE TO SEIZURE BEHAVIOR

Here's another frightening scenario: Imagine you're walking down the street when you're suddenly overcome by a complex partial seizure that causes you to speak incoherently, get drowsy and appear intoxicated. A frightened bystander calls 911, and when the police arrive they arrest you for drunk and disorderly conduct. You aren't even aware of what's happening until you suddenly "awaken" and realize that a police officer is leading you to his patrol car. You frantically try to explain that you were having a seizure, but the police ignore you. And as you're being taken to the police station, booked and put in a holding tank, you tell everyone you see that if you don't get your medicine (which is at home), you might have another seizure. No one seems too interested.

There are many documented cases of people who are arrested because their seizures are misinterpreted as illegal behavior. Some are taken into custody and charged with drunk and disorderly behavior, creating a riot, or committing an offense against public decency. Even worse, law enforcement personnel may mismanage seizures, leading to injury and in some rare cases, death.

You can protect yourself in the following ways:

- Always wear a Medic-Alert bracelet or necklace and show it to the authorities as soon as possible.

- Always carry a letter from your doctor explaining that you have epilepsy and describing your customary symptoms or if this is not available, an index card with all the information police might need to know.

- Alert your local police department to the fact that you have a seizure disorder and explain what your seizures look like and the types of behavior you exhibit.

- When possible carry your medications in the original containers rather than in an unmarked one.

- Let local law enforcement personnel know that there may be training available regarding the understanding and correct management of seizures. Training may be provided by your local chapter of the Epilepsy Foundation of America or a local advocacy group such as Epilepsy Life Links (www.epilepsylifelinks.com).

For more information see:

- **Jeanne A. Carpenter Epilepsy Legal Defense Fund**
  http://www.epilepsyfoundation.org/epilepsylegal/

- **Legal Services Corporation for State-by-State Resources**
  http://www.lsc.gov/

- **National Legal Aid Defense Fund**
  http://www.nlada.org/Defender

DENIED AFFORDABLE HEALTH INSURANCE

Finding affordable insurance is, to say the least, a challenge for people with epilepsy. Many insurance carriers either refuse coverage, citing a pre-existing condition, or charge such an exorbitant amount for premiums or deductibles that their policies are unaffordable. The same problems apply to automobile and life insurance, both of which can be difficult to find for those with epilepsy.

If you are working, the best health insurance may be the policy available through your employer. It's generally a group plan that you can join without having to worry about pre-existing coverage or additional charges.

However, the situation will be made more confusing by the soon-to-be-implemented regulations that are part of the larger new health care program. No one is quite sure how these changes will play out or which new rules will apply. To make matters more confusing, while the federal laws apply in every state, each state has its own set of additional regulations. All of this means that you will have to do a fair amount of research to find health insurance that offers you good coverage at an affordable price. Here are some websites that can help you in your search:

- **US Government Guide to Understanding Health Insurance** http://www.usa.gov/Citizen/Topics/Health/HealthInsurance.shtml

- **The Health Insurance Portability & Accountability Act of 1996 (HIPAA)**
  (protects you against insurance denial) http://www.cms.gov/HealthInsReformforConsume/02_WhatHIPAADoesandDoesNotDo.asp#TopOfPage

- **Comprehensive Omnibus Benefits Reform Act of 1986 (COBRA)**
  (assures you will have a temporary continuation of health coverage at group rates following the loss of employment)
- http://www.dol.gov/ebsa/cobra.html

- **The Patient Protection and Affordable Care Act**
  http://www.kff.org/healthreform/upload/8061.pdf

- **Automobile and Life Insurance Regulations**
  http://www.aiadc.org/aiapub/

Medicare

If you are 65 years or older, or less than 65 but have certain disabilities, you can qualify for Medicare, the federal government's own health insurance program. You'll find information on Medicare at:

- **Medicare Basics**
  http://www.medicare.gov/navigation/medicare-basics/medicare-basics-overview.aspx

- **Medicare Eligibility** http://www.medicare.gov/MedicareEligibility/Home.asp?dest=NAV|Home|GeneralEnrollment#TabTop

Medicaid

While the U.S. government provides Medicare, the states have a similar program called Medicaid that offers direct payment to your health care providers. Low-income families and their children, seniors, and people with disabilities are eligible. Each state has its own set of criteria for eligibility, including age, disability, income, net worth and US citizenship. For more information see:

- **Medicaid Basics**
  http://www.cms.gov/MedicaidGenInfo/

- **Medicaid Eligibility** http://www.cms.gov/MedicaidEligibility/02_AreYouEligible_.asp#TopOfPage

- **State-by-State Information** http://www.cms.gov/MedicaidEligibility/downloads/ListStateMedicaidWebsites.pdf

FINANCIAL DISTRESS DUE TO EPILEPSY

There is no denying that living with epilepsy and its consequences can take a toll on personal finances. For some, the biggest problem is unemployment or underemployment. But even if you have a steady job, the medical bills, loss of time from work, and use of vacation time and personal time for medical appointments can put a strain on your finances.

Fortunately, the government offers assistance programs. Chief among these is Social Security Disability Insurance (SSDI).

Social Security Disability Insurance (SSDI)

A seizure disorder may be considered a disabling condition but there are certain stipulations. As the Social Security Administration website explains: "Social Security pays benefits to people who cannot work because they have a medical condition that is expected to last at least one year or result in death. Federal law requires this very strict definition of disability."

To qualify for SSDI, you must provide basic information about yourself and your condition to the Social Security Administration. They will contact your doctors for additional information and apply various "can you work?" tests to determine whether or not you are eligible.

Adults with a documented disability may receive Social Security benefits after the age of 18. They must have worked in the past for a certain period of time in order to qualify, with the minimum number of work years depending on the individual's age. The disability must also prohibit performance of any kind of work. And it must have already lasted for at least one year, or be expected to last at least one year, or be expected to result in death. For more information, see:

- **The Adult Disability Starter Kit-Fact Sheet** http://www. ssa.gov/disability/disability_starter_kits_adult_factsheet. htm#disability
  To apply online:
  http://www.socialsecurity.gov/applyfor**disability**

Children with a documented disability may receive Social Security benefits until they reach the age of 18. In order to qualify, the child must have a disability that severely limits activity, and it must have lasted, or be expected to last, at least one year. To learn more, see:

- **The Child Disability Starter Kit** http://www.ssa.gov/disability/disability_starter_kits_child_eng.htm
  To apply online:
  www.ssa.gov/applyfordisability/child.htm

Supplemental Security Income (SSI)

A separate program, called Supplemental Security Income (SSI), provides money to adults who are disabled and have a low income or few resources. For more information, see:

- **Supplemental Security Income (SSI)**
  http://www.ssa.gov/pubs/11000.html

EXCLUDED FROM PARTICIPATING IN SCHOOL ACTIVITIES

There are two laws that protect your child's right to receive a free, appropriate education in spite of his or her disabilities: Section 504 of the Rehabilitation Act of 1973 and The Individual with Disabilities Education Act (IDEA).

Section 504 was designed to make sure that no one is excluded from participating in federally funded programs or activities because of a disability. This means that accommodations must be made to ensure the child's access to the learning environment and academic success.

IDEA ensures that a child with one or more of 13 specific disabilities receives special instruction and related services in the least restrictive environment (including a regular classroom whenever possible).

Both require that a plan be filed. For children who are *not* in need of specialized instruction, it's the 504 plan. For those who *do* need specialized instruction (this is the category covered by IDEA), it's the Individual Education Plan (IEP).

504 Plan

If your child has epilepsy and is attending elementary, secondary or post-secondary schooling, you'll need to file a 504 plan to help ensure that he/she can participate fully in all school activities and educational programs. The law requires every school to have a Section 504 coordinator, and you should work with this coordinator, as well as the school nurse, teachers, the principal, and/or other support staff, to develop the plan. The 504 plan should contain a list of all accommodations that must be made regarding your child's disability (e.g. special seating, an extra set of books to keep at home, wheelchair ramps, tape recorder and so on).

Participating in gym and going along on field trips can pose special problems for children with epilepsy. Talk with your treatment team about any sports/gym/travel restrictions that they feel should be put in place. Then, have your doctor draft a letter of explanation about these limitations to have on file with the school nurse and/or added to your child's 504 plan. Remember, your child's participation in these activities is protected by law. You have the right to request a special accommodation that will allow your child to share in all of these activities whenever possible.

- **Section 504 of the Rehabilitation Act of 1973**
  http://www.hhs.gov/ocr/civilrights/resources/factsheets/504.pdf

- **Section 504 Accommodation Plan - Sample**
  http://98.129.194.75//docs/Sample_504.pdf

- **Section 504 Accommodations for College Students**
  http://www.wrightslaw.com/info/sec504.college.accoms.brown.htm

- **Section 504 and ADA: Discrimination**
  http://www2.ed.gov/about/offices/list/ocr/504faq.html

- **Section 504 and ADA: Education of Children with Disabilities** http://www2.ed.gov/about/offices/list/ocr/504faq.html

Individualized Education Plan (IEP)

A small number of students with disabilities need significant assistance and remediation in school. They must work at their own pace and they require special instruction, different teaching methods and a change in curriculum in order to succeed. For these children, an Individualized Education Plan (IEP) must be filed. The IEP includes reasonable learning goals for the child and lists the services the school district needs to provide. Like the 504 plan, the IEP is created by you (the parent), the teachers involved (regular and special education), and/or other support staff. For more information, see:

- **Wrights Law - a complete guide to education law including the IEP process**
  http://wrightslaw.com

- **A Guide to the Individualized Education Program**
  http://ed.gov/parents/needs/speced/iepguide/index.html

Sometimes parents may need to consider the option of an advocate to join them in a meeting if they feel they are having trouble communicating all the child's needs and obtaining the necessary services. Many local Epilepsy Foundations have educators who can help. Our own Epilepsy Life Links also provides support to parents usually through one of neuropsychologists. In those cases, the doctor calls in during the IEP meeting to go over specific recommendations and key issues that should be considered. Parents who have experienced this are typically very happy with the results.

DON'T BE SHY!

The main reason that people fail to utilize the legal and financial protections offered by the government is they don't know about them. And even if they do, they are often embarrassed;

don't want to "make a scene" or feel unable to handle the details by themselves.

I urge you to remember that the best way to deal with epilepsy is to embrace life and live it to the fullest in every possible way. The legal and financial assistance outlined in this chapter is available so you can do just that. Reach out – ask for help – and accept whatever is offered. By accepting the good and positive things life has to offer, you (or your child) will become stronger and healthier, both physically and emotionally.

CHAPTER FIFTEEN
COPING STRATEGIES FOR FAMILIES AND FRIENDS

As you undoubtedly know by now, a diagnosis of epilepsy creates huge challenges for both family and close friends of the patient. Accepting the diagnosis is the first hurdle; understanding the disorder is the second. The third step – learning to live a normal life in spite of the ever-present fear of seizures, endless doctor appointments, school issues, sibling issues, work issues, transportation issues – can be nothing short of overwhelming. You may find yourself wondering, "Will life ever be normal again?"

The families and friends of my patients always have many questions that they need to have answered, especially soon after diagnosis. They want to know what to do, how to act, what to say, how to make the patient safe, how to handle seizures, and so on. The aim of this chapter is to address some of those common questions to give you a place to start helping your family member or friend. As always, the treating neurologist/epileptologist should be your primary source of information. Then, learn all you can about the disorder by reading books (like this one) and visiting the websites listed in Appendix 1 – Epilepsy Resources and elsewhere throughout the book.

Let's start with the most frequently asked question: What do you do when someone has a seizure?

WHAT DO I DO IF I'M WITH SOMEONE WHO HAS A SEIZURE?

Perhaps the greatest concern that family members and close friends have is how to handle a seizure in progress. What do you do? How do you act? Should you restrain the person? Should you call 911?

The general guidelines are:

- Stay calm *Seizures start and end without intervention most of the time. *Be reassuring but don't hold the person down

- Protect the person from injury and dangerous objects that are near. (For example, if someone falls on the street, remove nearby rocks or sharp objects.)

- Look at your watch and start timing the seizure as soon as it starts so you can report this to the doctor. (Certain medications may be necessary to abort a prolonged seizure, which is usually defined as two minutes or longer.)

- Loosen tight neckwear, ties, scarves, etc.

- If the person has fallen, turn on his or her side and put something soft under the head to prevent injury.

- Never put anything in the person's mouth, and never hold the person down. (You can lose your finger that way! And, contrary to popular belief, the tongue will never be "swallowed.")

- Look for ID bracelet or card
- Stay with the person until the seizure is over and they are recovered.

In most cases, calling for emergency medical assistance is not necessary; however, if you have any doubts, do not hesitate to call 911. If calling 911 doesn't seem necessary, once the person has recovered enough to be able to walk, take him or her home to rest. Be sure to call the doctor and report the seizure, including the time it lasted and the symptoms.

When to call 911?

> The seizure lasts more than 2 minutes
> There is no ID specifying that the person suffers from epilepsy
> The person is not waking up or is having difficulty breathing after the seizure
> The woman is pregnant
> The person has injured him/herself during the seizure
> The seizure occurred in water

FREQUENTLY ASKED QUESTIONS

In my 23 years of treating epilepsy, I've been asked literally thousands of questions by the friends and families of people with epilepsy. I've included some of the most common ones below as a place for you to start. You'll undoubtedly have others, so be sure to ask the epileptologist or another member of the medical team about anything that confuses or troubles you.

Q: What is the best way to tell my daughter about her epilepsy
A: It will depend on her age and ability to understand but it can help to start by drawing a picture of a brain. You can show her that there is a part of her brain that lights up when she has a seizure. Explain that the doctor is giving her medication to help stop this from happening and that is one of the reasons it is so important she take her medications every day.

There are several well-written books for children of different ages in which the characters have epilepsy and deal with different challenges. You can read some of these together.

Q: *I am a mother of a 3 year old boy and I have epilepsy. Should I start talking to my son now about my epilepsy or will it just scare him unnecessarily?*

A: *In the event that your child witnesses one of your seizures, the more he knows about what they look like and what steps he can take, the more likely he is to feel in control of the situation and the less frightening the memory will be. It is never too early to begin teaching a child about 911, your first and last name and your address. You may also want to put your emergency contact on speed dial and teach him how to dial out. You may also teach him one or two small first aid activities he can do (i.e. put a pillow under mom's head when it is over, stay with mom until the seizure is over). Also remind him that although the seizure may be scary,* <u>mom will be alright</u>*.*

Q: *My newborn has been having neonatal seizures. I'm reluctant to tell my parents and family about this because I don't want to worry them. Should I keep it to myself?*

A: You might think that sheltering your parents and family from news of their new family member's epilepsy is an act of kindness. But family members who eventually find out may feel isolated, hurt and excluded. Almost all of them would rather know so that they can do something to help and they may in fact be able to provide you with useful emotional support. Consider making them a part of your team. You may also obtain useful family medical history by talking about this to them.

Q *My child has Lennox-Gastaut syndrome and sometimes I get completely overwhelmed when caring for him. Where do I look for help?*

A. Caring for a child with epilepsy is a huge challenge that can easily become isolating and overwhelming. It's essential to your own health and well being that you put together an effective support network, beginning with your treatment team. Extended family and friends may be able to give you some time off, provide transportation, help with household chores and give emotional support. There are also respite programs through foundations and governmental agencies in some areas. If your child qualifies, he/she will be cared for by a trained caretaker and you will have a set number of hours for yourself and your chores.

The federal government sponsors early intervention programs for infants and toddlers with disabilities that not only support the child, but the entire family as well. Program components that you may find useful include:

- family education and counseling

- home visits

- parent support groups

- vision services

- speech pathology and audiology

- occupational therapy

- assistive technology devices and services

- physical therapy

- psychological services

- nursing services

- nutrition services

- social work services

For more information, visit the following U.S. Department of Education website:

- **Early Intervention for Infants and Toddlers with Disabilities** http://www2.ed.gov/programs/osepeip/index.html

Q. Sometimes it seems that my child's epilepsy is the focal point of everything we do in our family. It's tough on everybody. What can we do about this?

A. It's critical that you keep epilepsy from undermining the well-being of the rest of the family. Here are some tips for maintaining balance:

- **Communicate**. Make sure that everyone in the family has a chance to express their fears regarding the family member with epilepsy, learn about epilepsy, and voice their disappointment, frustration, and possible misplaced guilt about changes in family dynamics. Attending a support group for patients and their loved ones is often valuable.

- **Prioritize**. Place as much importance on scheduling family activities as you would on setting up a medical appointment. Both are vital to family health.

- **Preserve family health.** Neglecting your health and the health of the rest of the family is easy to do when so much time is consumed by one person's medical condition. Keep in mind that if you become ill, you may not be able to care for your family member. Foster a healthy lifestyle for your family that includes proper diet, exercise, and regular checkups.

- **Recognize trouble**. At the first sign of a problem, look for help. Speak up to your treatment team. They have seen many families like yours and may have a number of treatment recommendations for you. Many families dealing with the challenges of epilepsy benefit from family and/or individual psychotherapy.

Q. I'd like to enroll my child in pre-school even though her seizures are not well-controlled. Do you have any suggestions as to what kind of pre-school I should look for?

A. When a young child has seizures, safety and special programs aimed at meeting developmental milestones are the most important parts of any program. Special education at the pre-school level may be provided for free through your local school district, following evaluation of your child's needs. If special education services are not needed, look for a program that emphasizes the acceptance of differences and the optimization of abilities. Then educate the program staff as to how to recognize your child's seizures and provide appropriate first aid.

Q. My daughter, who has benign rolandic epilepsy, is about to start elementary school. She has only had a few seizures and all of them happened at night while she was sleeping. She takes no medication. Do I need to tell the school about this?

A. While not disclosing her condition will afford your child privacy, disclosure will ensure the highest level of safety. You should bear in mind that asking your child to keep the seizures a secret may make her feel that she has something to hide. This could lower her self-esteem and create feelings of guilt. Only you know what is the best decision and who may be the key persons in school with whom you could share this information comfortably.

Q. Can I assume that teachers are trained in the handling of epileptic seizures?

A. Absolutely not. And new regulations added to the Health Insurance Portability and Accountability Act (**HIPAA**) prevent the school nurse from disclosing your child's epilepsy to *anyone*, including his or her teachers. So *you* will need to inform the teachers and school support staff about your child's condition and any first aid you would like them to offer. The support staff could include bus drivers, lunchroom workers, and playground monitors. Arranging for first aid training of all of the above might prove very helpful. You could arrange to have a local epilepsy foundation or patient advocacy group invited to your child's school to provide education on seizure recognition (not all seizures look alike) and first aid.

Q. Should we talk to the other children in the classroom about my son's seizures, or is it better just to let sleeping dogs lie?
A. It depends on your son. Some children with epilepsy have an open attitude about their seizures and would like to participate in classroom instruction about epilepsy. Such training can be provided to children of all ages and will underscore the idea that everyone is different in some way, and those differences should be accepted in the most positive light. Other children would prefer not to share their epilepsy with their peers. Their reasons for this could be explored and should be respected.

Q. My 7 year-old son has behavior problems and gets in trouble regularly at school. Is this typical of children with benign rolandic epilepsy?
A. Epilepsy is not necessarily associated with disruptive behavior. Every behavior has a cause; it may be anger, frustration, fear, peer rejection, bullying or even medication side effects. Working closely with your treatment team and teacher/school support staff may help you uncover the cause and find a remedy. Since behavioral issues can be a significant barrier to educational success, they need to be addressed quickly.

Q. My daughter, who has childhood absence epilepsy, is struggling in school. I'd like to get her evaluated to see if medication side effects are part of the problem. How do I go about this?
A. Children with epilepsy are at greater risk of developing learning disabilities and weaknesses in attention, concentration, memory and

language. It is extremely important that a thorough psychoeducational evaluation be done as soon as these concerns arise, so classroom and teaching accommodations can be made quickly. As a parent, you have a legal right to obtain such an evaluation of your child through the school district's special education department. To start the process, visit:

- **National Dissemination Center for Children With Disabilities**
  http://www.nichcy.org/Pages/StateSpecificInfo.aspx
  (Then click on: your state; Special Education; Laws, Regulations & Policies; and type in the search box: psycho-educational evaluation.)

Some parents choose to go to an independent neuropsychologist who specializes in pediatric epilepsy for an "objective" viewpoint. The report with recommendations can be submitted to the school and the doctor can be present (in person or on the phone) at the school meetings to help facilitate decision-making regarding any necessary accommodations.

Q. How can I make sure my child gets the best possible education, in spite of her epilepsy?
A. First, it's important that you develop realistic educational goals based on past performance and up-to-date evaluations. Then, do the following:

- Take the time to know and appreciate education law, so you will understand your child's rights and the school's responsibilities. (See http://wrightslaw.com)

- Find out exactly what the school has to offer in the way of programs and disability services.

- Be prepared with supporting documentation when meeting with teachers, special education departments, and school officials to request special accommodations for your child.

- Enlist the support of an educational advocate when you feel that you need help.

Q. My husband thinks I'm overprotective of our 15 year-old son who has juvenile myoclonic epilepsy. But for me, safety is a number one priority. How can I keep our son safe without smothering him?

A. Balancing safety with independence can be tricky but it's absolutely necessary if your child is to become a self-reliant, responsible adult. To do so, you must understand the safety risks associated with his particular type of epilepsy. Then you'll need to differentiate between the activities he truly needs to avoid and those he can engage in with minimal to some risk. Talk to your child's medical team about your concerns, and offer your child an opportunity to discuss activities and restrictions directly with the doctor or epilepsy nurse. This may help put him on the road to making reasonable choices. Remember, as your child grows the shift towards independence will move and you, as parents, and your son will need to make further adjustments.

Q. My son has juvenile myoclonic epilepsy, which requires a lot of my time and attention. My other children resent this and act up a lot. What should I do?

A. Siblings of children with epilepsy often feel neglected, jealous of the attention the ailing child receives, and angry about the family lifestyle changes that accompany this diagnosis. Having frank conversations with the siblings about the changes they are seeing, creating a "special time" for each, and engaging in some family therapy can help change attitudes and solve problems. Sometimes local epilepsy foundations run sibling support groups that your children may benefit from attending. You may also consider involving the whole family in positive epilepsy activities (i.e. epilepsy walk, fund raiser).

Q. My daughter really wants to participate in gymnastics but that's not possible because of her seizures. How do I handle this?

A. Offer alternatives. There are going to be times when your child will want to participate in an activity that is risky. Anticipate this and be ready with other options. Perhaps she could get take dance classes or some other form of movement that doesn't involve flying around parallel bars or vaulting over a horse. Recognize and foster her abilities. If she's good in art, for example, build on that strength. It will increase her self-esteem and may help her find her place in life without putting her safety at risk. Be creative and you'll likely find several leisure activities she will enjoy that won't involve a safety risk.

Of course, there will be times when she will push the boundaries and fall on her face. But don't we all? That's how we learn about the negative consequences of bad choices. Try your best to be protective but not to be overprotective as hard as that may be.

Q. Is the onset of menstruation a cause of epilepsy?

A. Although some types of epilepsy, such as juvenile myoclonic and juvenile absence, may start about the same time that menstruation first begins, menstruation itself does not cause epilepsy. However, catamenial seizures are associated with it, increasing the likelihood of seizures during the two weeks leading up to the menstrual period. Ask your epileptologist or gynecologist for more information if the seizures seem to occur repeatedly at the same time of the month.

Q. Should I get involved in making sure my husband takes his antiseizure medications? Or is it his responsibility?

A. Seizure control is highly dependent on taking the proper amount of the proper medication at the proper times. (See Chapter 6 – Medication for more information.) If the patient was your child, obviously you would provide the medication and make sure he took it. But with an adult, there's a fine line between reminding and nagging. If you feel your husband is likely to forget to take the medication, you should provide gentle reminders. You may be able to help him by providing him with an electronic device with an alarm or a pill box. In these ways, you can help him without being in his business every day.

Q. My new friend just told me she has epilepsy. Should I ask her to tell me more about it or basically ignore it?
A. In general, you should treat a person with epilepsy the same way you would want to be treated if the situation were reversed. You would want your friends to treat you the same way they always have, be supportive and helpful when you need help, yet allow you to be independent whenever possible. In short, treat your friend as normally as possible.

If you have questions about how the disorder affects her, ask her in a thoughtful and caring manner. No need to tiptoe around: going straight to the source will help you understand the situation better and increase the feeling of intimacy between the two of you. You might ask:

- Do you have frequent seizures, or do the seizures rarely occur?

- How long have you had seizures?

- Can you drive?

- Can you work?

- What are the side effects of the medications you take?

- How often do you need to take your medications?

- What are your seizures like?

- How long do your seizures last?

- What can I do for you?

- What would you like me to do if you have a seizure?

Q. Are there any other ways that I support my friend?
A. Some medications cause reactions when combined with certain foods (e.g., grapefruit), other medications, birth control pills, and/or alcohol. Ask your friend what she needs to avoid and support her in her efforts. For example, if she needs to avoid alcohol, suggest activities that you can do together that don't involve drinking.

Q. My grandson is about to graduate from high school with a special education diploma. Is it true that he won't be accepted to any college?
A. In most states, the minimal requirement for entrance into college is a General Educational Development (GED) diploma. If your grandson truly wants to go to college, he should look into getting a GED first. If not, trade school may be good option.

As for which college or trade school to choose, key epilepsy factors will be seizure control, ability to drive or take public transportation, and the capacity to live safely away from home. When living on campus, plenty of help is available. In a dormitory setting, for example, the Residential Advisor (RA) and roommates can be trained in seizure recognition and first aid. Special assistance programs on campus may include tutoring, developmental education programs, study groups, and math, writing and/or reading labs. The special services department may also offer help in the form of note takers, readers, time extensions for tests and papers, classroom/computer adaptations and audio-taped materials.

For more information, see:

- **Accommodations for College Students:**
  http://www.wrightslaw.com/info/sec504.college.accoms.brown.htm

- **Services for students with disabilities:**
  http://www.collegeboard.com/ssd/student/index.html

- **Trade school information:**
  http://www.collegesurfing.com/content/cat/trade/446

CHAPTER SIXTEEN
YOU *CAN* LIVE A NORMAL LIFE!

With the diagnosis of epilepsy comes change. For awhile, the "can do" list becomes shorter while the "can't do" list seems to grow by leaps and bounds... especially right after the initial diagnosis. Adjusting your mind and body to a different lifestyle will require patience, courage, education, the assistance of family, friends and community, and plenty of hard work. (And did I mention *patience?*) It's important that you understand that change is necessary, and that change can be positive. But it will take time to normalize. The more you understand about epilepsy and how it affects every aspect of your life, the better prepared you will be to make the necessary adjustments. In the end, I think you'll find that your lifetime goals may be a bit redirected, but they can be achieved.

I began this book by saying that epilepsy is a frightening disorder. And indeed it is. But you now know a great deal about the causes and types of seizures, the medicines and diets that help control them, how to resolve associated legal and social issues, and much more. You are also aware of the many forms of assistance that are available, and know where you can obtain that help.

Because of your newly found knowledge, you are much better equipped now to understand epilepsy, communicate with your physician and the other members of your health team, and successfully handle the many accompanying health, family, social and legal issues.

You are well prepared to turn distress into success, gain control of your epilepsy, and lead a healthy, productive and fulfilling life.

There's only one more thing you need: the resolve to live life to its fullest, in the safest possible manner. This means following the guidelines set by your doctor and treatment team, while casting aside any ideas that you are "damaged" or "less" than other people. I've seen too many patients who were afraid to spread their wings, even after their seizures were under excellent control. They continued to restrict their activities, hold back on forming new relationships and, in general, set their goals too low. I urge you to dream great dreams and strive to make them come true. You are worth it.

At the beginning of Chapter 2, I named certain people who had accomplished great things in spite of their epilepsy. To that list, we can add Alexander the Great, Pope Pius IX, the great Russian composer Tchaikovsky, Chief Justice of the U.S. Supreme Court John Roberts, inventor Alfred Nobel, poet Lord Byron, novelist Dostoyevsky, Bud Abbot of Abbot & Costello, actor Danny Glover and composer George Frederick Handel. And there are many, many others whose names you wouldn't recognize who have led wonderful, productive lives and made a difference.

They didn't let epilepsy stop them, and neither should you. You *can* control epilepsy, and lead a healthy, happy and fulfilling life. It's within your grasp!

APPENDIX 1
EPILEPSY RESOURCES

GENERAL INFORMATION

The treating epileptologist/neurologist is your best source of information, but if you feel you need more, be wary of general search engine results. There are literally thousands of websites that offer explanations and advice regarding epilepsy, but you should examine them carefully and not "trust" them without reading them carefully. Here are some that I recommend (see below). Remember that misinformation can easily lead to mismanagement of epilepsy. Below is a list of reliable websites:

- **Northeast Regional Epilepsy Group**
  http://www.epilepsygroup.com/epilepsy-information5-59/epilepsy-information.htm
- **American Academy of Neurology Patient Materials**
  http://www.aan.com/go/practice/patient
- **American Epilepsy Society**
  http://www.aesnet.org/
- **American Neurological Association** http://www.aneuroa.org/i4a/pages/index.cfm?pageid=1
- **Brave Kids**
  http://www.bravekids.org/
- **Epilepsy Advocate**
  http://www.epilepsyadvocate.com/about-epilepsy/types-of-seizures.aspx

- **Epilepsy Foundation** http://epilepsyfoundation.org/about-epilepsy/whatisepilepsy/index.cfm
- **Epilepsy Life Links** www.epilepsylifelinks.com
- **International League Against Epilepsy** http://www.ilae-epilepsy.org/Visitors/Centre/Brochuresforchapters.cfm
- **MedlinePlus** http://www.nlm.nih.gov/medlineplus/epilepsy.html
- National Institute of Neurological Disorders and Stroke http://www.ninds.nih.gov/disorders/epilepsy/epilepsy.htm

INFORMATION ABOUT SPECIFIC CONDITIONS

- **Autism Speaks** http://www.autismspeaks.org/about_us.php
- **Brain Injury Association of America** http://www.biausa.org/
- **Dravet Syndrome** http://www.idea-league.org/
- Intractable Childhood Epilepsy Alliance http://www.ice-epilepsy.org/
- **Lennox-Gastaut Syndrome Foundation** http://www.lgsfoundation.org/
- National Organization for Rare Diseases http://www.rarediseases.org/
- **Tuberous Sclerosis Alliance** http://www.tsalliance.org

MEDICATION

General Information
- **National Library of Medicine Drug Information Database** http://www.nlm.nih.gov/medlineplus/druginformation.html

- **RxList**
  http://www.rxlist.com/script/main/hp.asp

Miscellaneous
- **Adverse Event Reporting Program (FDA)**
  http://www.fda.gov/Safety/MedWatch/default.htm
- **Information on New Drugs (FDA)**
  http://www.fda.gov/Drugs/DrugSafety/
  PostmarketDrugSafetyInformationforPatientsandProviders/
  UCM111085
- **Nutrition & Epilepsy Drugs – Drug/Nutrient Interaction**
  http://www.healingwithnutrition.com/edisease/epilepsy/epi-lepsydrugs.html

Free or Low-Cost Medication
- **Rx Assist**
  http://www.rxassist.org
- Prescription Assistance
  http://epilepsylifelinks.com/services_patient-assistance-pro-grams.php

RESEARCH

- **Citizens United for Research in Epilepsy (CURE)**
  http://www.cureepilepsy.org/research/
- **Epilepsy Foundation**
  http://www.epilepsyfoundation.org/research/
- **National Institutes of Neurological Diseases and Stroke Research Page**
  http://www.ninds.nih.gov/research/epilepsyweb/index.htm
- **Northeast Regional Epilepsy Group Research**
  http://epilepsygroup.com/clinical-detail4-10-15/epilepsy-research-treatment-drug-trials.htm

EDUCATION

General

- **Accommodations for College Students**
  http://www.wrightslaw.com/info/sec504.college.accoms.brown.htm
- **College Board Services for Students with Disabilities**
  http://www.collegeboard.com/ssd/student/index.html
- **Epilepsy Foundation - IDEA Q & A**
  http://www.epilepsyfoundation.org/resources/epilepsy/legal/loader.cfm?csModule=security/getfile&pageid=36485
- **Epilepsy Foundation – Expanding Understanding of Epilepsy in U. S. Schools** http://www.epilepsyfoundation.org/resources/newsroom/pressreleases/Discovery-Education-and-Epilepsy-Foundation-Partner-to-Expand-Understanding-of-Epilepsy-in-US-Schools.cfm)
- **IDEA - Individuals with Disabilities Education Act**
  http://idea.ed.gov/
- **National Center for Learning Disabilities** (includes information for college students)
  http://www.ncld.org/
- **Northeast Regional Epilepsy Group Cognitive (Neuropsychological) Services** http://www.epilepsygroup.com/diagnostic-detail4-11-9/epilepsy-diagnosis-memory-neuropsychology.htm
- **Office of Special Education and Rehabilitative Services**
  http://www2.ed.gov/about/offices/list/osers/osep/index.html
- **Special Education Resources for Children with Disabilities** http://www.nichcy.org/Pages/StateSpecificInfo.aspx (Look under "Disability - Specific Organizations" then click on your state.)
- **Trade School Information**
  http://www.collegesurfing.com/ce/search/?campaign_id=12619420

Rights

- **Epilepsy Foundation - Elementary and Secondary Education Law** http://www.epilepsyfoundation.org/living-withepilepsy/educators/educationlaws/elementary-and-secondary-education-law.cfm
- **IDEA: Individuals with Disabilities Education Act** http://idea.ed.gov
- **IDEA: Q & A** http://www.epilepsyfoundation.org/resources/epilepsy/legal/loader.cfm?csModule=security/getfile&pageid=36485
- **IEP – US Department of Education Guide to the Individualized Education Programs** http://ed.gov/parents/needs/speced/iepguide/index.html
- **US Department of Education Factsheet on Section 504 of the Rehabilitation Act of 1973** http://www.hhs.gov/ocr/civilrights/resources/factsheets/504.pdf
- **Section 504 Accommodation Plan - Sample** http://98.129.194.75//docs/Sample_504.pdf
- **Section 504 Accommodations for College Students** http://www.wrightslaw.com/info/sec504.college.accoms.brown.htm
- **Section 504: Protecting Students With Disabilities** http://www2.ed.gov/about/offices/list/ocr/504faq.html
- **Wright's Law** (a complete guide to education law including the IEP process) http://wrightslaw.com/

FUNDING & SCHOLARSHIPS

Scholarships, grants for summer camp, funding for tuition, school supplies and living expenses, financial aid for specific disabilities and seizure alert dogs are available to those in need. See the websites below, but also check with your local Epilepsy Foundation affiliate to get updates and find out about selection criteria.

General

- **US Department of Education: Education Resource Organizations Directory** http://wdcrobcolp01.ed.gov/Programs/EROD/org_list.cfm?category_ID=SHE
- **Federal Student Aid: General Information on Federal Student Aid Programs** www.fafsa.ed.gov
- **National Center for Learning Disabilities** www.ncld.org

Summer Camp Scholarships and Camps

- **Northeast Regional Epilepsy Group Camp Scholarship Program** http://www.epilepsylifelinks.com/scholarship-children-adults.php
- **UCB scholarships** *http://www.ucbepilepsyscholarship.com/*
- **Summer camps for children with epilepsy and scholarship opportunities** *http://epilepsytalk.com/2011/02/11/epilepsy-summer-camps/*

Disability-Related Scholarships and Awards

- **Alexis Buskirk Memorial Book Scholarship** (for students at the University of Alaska at Anchorage) http://www.eastchance.com/scholarship.asp?id=6960
- **Foundation for Science and Disability** www.as.wvu.edu/-scidis/organize/fsdinfo.html
- **Incight Go-Getter Scholarships and Awards** http://www.incight.org/
- **Project Vision: A Bilingual Website for Youth with Disabilities** http://www.proyectovision.net/english/opportunities/grants.html
- **Northeast Regional Epilepsy Group college/trade school scholarship Program** http://www.epilepsylifelinks.com/scholarship-children-adults.php

Seizure Assistance Dogs

Dogs can be trained to get help, push life-alert buttons, retrieve phones and help/comfort a person during a seizure. These organizations train these special dogs and provide them at no cost to those in need.

- **Paws With a Cause**
  www.pawswithacause.org
- **Assistance Dogs International**
  http://www.assistancedogsinternational.org
- **Canine Assistance**
  www.canineassistants.org

Disability or Supplemental Security Income

- **The Adult Disability Starter Kit-Fact Sheet** http://www.
  ssa.gov/disability/disability_starter_kits_adult_factsheet.
  htm#disability.
  To apply online:
- http://www.socialsecurity.gov/applyfordisability.
- **The Child Disability Starter Kit** http://www.ssa.gov/dis-
  ability/disability_starter_kits_child_eng.htm
  To apply online:
- www.ssa.gov/applyfordisability/child.htm
- **Supplemental Security Income (SSI)**
  http://www.ssa.gov/pubs/11000.html

Medicare/Medicaid

- **Medicare Basics** http://www.medicare.gov/navigation/medi-
  care-basics/medicare-basics-overview.aspx
- **Medicare Eligibility** http://www.medicare.gov/
  MedicareEligibility/Home.asp?dest=NAV|Home|GeneralEnr
  ollment#TabTop
- **Medicaid Basics** http://www.cms.gov/MedicaidGenInfo/
- **Medicaid General Overview Information**
  http://www.cms.gov/MedicaidGenInfo/
- **Medicaid Eligibility** http://www.cms.gov/
  MedicaidEligibility/02_AreYouEligible_.asp#TopOfPage

- Medicaid: State-by-State Information http://www.cms.gov/MedicaidEligibility/downloads/ListStateMedicaidWebsites.pdf

LEGAL RIGHTS

General

- ADA - Department of Justice Title III of the Americans with Disabilities Act
http://www.ada.gov/reg3a.html
- ADA Guide to Disabilities Rights Laws
http://www.ada.gov/cguide.htm
- Equal Employment Opportunity Commission (EEOC) – Disability Discrimination
http://www.eeoc.gov/laws/types/disability.cfm
- EEOC Fact Sheet: Questions and Answers About Epilepsy In the Workplace http://www.eeoc.gov/facts/epilepsy.html
- Epilepsy Foundation Fact Sheet: Discrimination by Public Accommodations and Federal Law
http://www.epilepsyfoundation.org/resources/epilepsy/loader.cfm?csModule=security/getfile&PageID=21494
- Epilepsy Foundation: Legal Rights, Legal Issues
http://www.epilepsyfoundation.org/resources/epilepsy/legal/loader.cfm?csModule=security/getfile&pageid=36451
- Epilepsy Foundation: Legal Rights of Persons with Epilepsy http://www.epilepsyfoundation.org/resources/epilepsy/legalfactsheets.cfm
- Section 504 of the Rehabilitation Act of 1973
http://www.hhs.gov/ocr/civilrights/resources/factsheets/504.pdf
- Section 504 and ADA: Protecting Students with Disabilities
http://www2.ed.gov/about/offices/list/ocr/504faq.html

Defense Funds
- **Jeanne A. Carpenter Epilepsy Legal Defense Fund**
  http://www.epilepsyfoundation.org/epilepsylegal/
- **Legal Services Corporation for State-by-State Resources**
  http://www.lsc.gov/
- **National Legal Aid Defense Fund**
  http://www.nlada.org/Defender

Insurance
- **US Government Guide to Understanding Health Insurance** http://www.usa.gov/Citizen/Topics/Health/HealthInsurance.shtml
- **The Health Insurance Portability & Accountability Act of 1996 (HIPAA)** (Protects you against insurance denial) http://www.cms.gov/HealthInsReformforConsume/02_WhatHIPAADoesandDoesNotDo.asp#TopOfPage
- **Comprehensive Omnibus Benefits Reform Act of 1986 (COBRA)** (Assures you will have temporary continuation of health coverage at group rates for a specific amount of time following loss of employment) http://www.dol.gov/ebsa/cobra.html
- **The Patient Protection and Affordable Care Act** http://www.kff.org/healthreform/upload/8061.pdf

PUBLIC TRANSPORTATION FOR PEOPLE WITH DISABILITIES

- **Paratransit Transportation: General Information** http://www.disability.gov/transportation
- **Paratransit Transportation: Eligibility Manual** http://ntl.bts.gov/DOCS/ada.html
- USA Public Transportation (State by State) http://www.publictransportation.org/Pages/default.aspx

For Veterans:

- **The National Resource Web Directory of National Public Transportation Services Available for Veterans**: https://www.nationalresourcedirectory.gov/transportation_and_travel (Click on "Transportation Assistance and Public Transportation")
- **The Disabled American Veterans Transportation Network** http://www.dav.org/volunteers/Ride.aspx

HOME SAFETY

- **Epilepsy Foundation - Home Safety** http://www.epilepsyfoundation.org/aboutepilepsy/healthrisks/homesafety.cfm

SUPPORT GROUPS

Attending a support group regularly may help you deal with the stressors and challenges of living with epilepsy. To find one in your area, visit:

- **Epilepsy Foundation Local Support (Directory of national epilepsy support groups)** http://www.epilepsyfoundation.org/aboutus/Find-an-Affiliate.cfm
- **Epilepsy Life Links (Free support groups in NY and NJ)** http://www.epilepsylifelinks.com/epilepsy-support-groups.php Ask your treatment team if they provide a support group in-house or if they recommend a support group nearby.

TRAVELING WITH EPILEPSY

- **Article on International Travel With Epilepsy** http://www.epilepsy.com/epilepsy/journal/issue1/intl_travel?gclid=CKKU_M7A3K0CFRZ3gwodUyfU6w
- **Epilepsy Foundation - Driving and Travel: Driver Information by State**

http://www.epilepsyfoundation.org/resources/drivin-gandtravel.cfm
- **Epilepsy Foundation - Tips on Traveling with a Child Who Has Epilepsy**
http://www.epilepsyfoundation.org/affiliates/massri/loader.cfm?csModule=security/getfile&pageid=28391
- **International Travel With Epilepsy**
http://www.epilepsy.com/epilepsy/journal/issue1/intl_travel?gclid=CKKU_M7A3K0CFRZ3gwodUyfU6w

WORKING WITH A DISABILITY

- **Americans with Disabilities Act**
http://www.ada.gov
- **Career Planning Page from Disabilty.gov**
https://www.disability.gov/employment/career_planning
- **Epilepsy Support - Employment**
http://www.epilepsylifelinks.com/services_employment.php
- **US Equal Employment Opportunity Commission – Disability Discrimination**
http://www.eeoc.gov/laws/types/disability.cfm
- **Epilepsy Foundation: Information on Military Service**
http://www.epilepsyfoundation.org/livingwithepilepsy/employmenttopics/safetysensitivejobs/militaryservice.cfm
- **Plan for Achieving Self Support (PASS)** (from the Social Security Administration)
http://www.ssa.gov/disabilityresearch/wi/pass.htm
- **Questions and Answers About Epilepsy in the Workplace and The Americans With Disabilities Act (US Equal Opportunity Commission)**
http://www.eeoc.gov/facts/epilepsy.html
- **Sample Resumes**
http://www.careeronestop.org/ResumeGuide/MoreSampleResumes.aspx

- **U.S. Department of Labor – One-Stop Career Centers** http://www.dol.gov/dol/topic/training/onestop.htm
- **Veterans Programs – Epilepsy Life Links** http://www.epilepsylifelinks.com/services_veterans.php
- **Veterans – What You Need to Know from the Epilepsy Foundation** http://www.epilepsyfoundation.org/resources/veterans.cfm
- **Workforce Investment Act Training Programs (Directory of programs by state)** http://www.careeronestop.org/WiaProviderSearch.asp
- **Working With a Disability and Employment Supports** https://www.disability.gov/employment/working_with_a_disability_%26_employment_supports
- **Workplace Rights of People with Epilepsy** (from the The U.S. Equal Employment Opportunity Commission) http://www.eeoc.gov/facts/epilepsy.html
- **Social Security-Ticket to Work Program** http://www.chooseworkttw.net/
- **Pregnancy Registries for anti epileptic medications** http://www.aedpregnancyregistry.org/

ADVOCACY - SPREADING THE WORD ABOUT EPILEPSY

Promoting epilepsy awareness is a good way to raise consciousness, connect with others, increase your knowledge, and help dispel the myths about epilepsy and those who have it. You can also write or email your government officials about epilepsy research funding, employment advocacy, medication switching (when a pharmacist can choose whether to give you the prescribed medication or replace it with a generic without the doctors consent) and many other issues that are currently before Congress or need to be introduced. These websites can help you find out how you can help spread the word:

Organizations Working to Increase Epilepsy Awareness
- **Epilepsy Foundation**
  http://epilepsyfoundation.org/advocacy/
- **Purple Day: March 26 is epilepsy awareness day**
  http://www.purpleday.org/
- **Epilepsy Lifel Lnks** http://www.epilepsylifelinks.com/volunteer.php
- **World Health Organization Global Campaign Against Epilepsy: Out of the Shadows** http://www.who.int/mental_health/management/globalepilepsycampaign/en/index.html
- **Danny Did Foundation**: Raises awareness about SUDEP http://www.dannydid.org/
- **SUDEP Aware** http://www.sudepaware.org/
- **Talk About It** http://www.talkaboutit.org/
- **Northeast Regional Epilepsy Group: Community Events and News** http://www.epilepsygroup.com/events-news-epilepsy-new-york-new-jersey-connecticut

Social Media (Facebook):
- Official Epilepsy Foundation of America and local affiliates
- Epilepsy Life Links
- Epilepsia en Latino America
- Epilepsy Foundation of America (E-communities*)*

Community Events/Fundraisers

Fundraising is an important part of the income for any agency, especially since grant monies are at a premium and governmental support is rapidly decreasing. Events can take the form of bowl-a-thons, galas, golf tournaments, Mardi Gras events or mud volleyball tournaments. There are fundraising walks sponsored by the National Epilepsy Foundation, Epilepsy Foundation affiliates, or private organizations. You'll find there are countless opportunities to make a difference. Get involved! The more you do, the more in charge you are!

APPENDIX 2
SEIZURE-RELATED DRIVING REGULATIONS LISTED BY STATE

STATE	REQUIRED PERIOD OF SEIZURE FREEDOM	REQUIREMENTS FOR REINSTATEMENT	REQUIRED UPDATES FOLLOWING REINSTATEMENT	PHYSICIAN REPORTING REQUIRED
ALABAMA	6 months (some exceptions apply)	Physician certification of fitness to drive must be submitted. An individual may be required to undergo a medical examination to determine whether they are able to safely operate a motor vehicle.	Periodic medical updates may be required at discretion of the DMV.	NO
ALASKA	6 months	Physician certification of fitness to drive must be submitted. No restricted or probationary licenses are available	Semi-annual neurological examinations may be required at discretion of DMV	NO

State	Seizure-free period	Requirements	Medical updates	Physician reporting
ARIZONA	3 months (some exceptions apply)	Physician certification of fitness to drive must be submitted. An individual who experiences a seizure must discontinue driving and undergo a medical examination to determine whether they are able to safely operate a motor vehicle.	Periodic medical updates may be required at discretion of DMV.	NO
ARKANSAS	12 months	Physician certification of fitness to drive must be submitted. No restricted or probationary licenses are available.	Periodic medical updates may be required at discretion of DMV.	NO
CALIFORNIA	3–6 months (some exceptions apply)	Physician certification of fitness to drive must be submitted. Diverse types of probationary periods are established based on episodes or lapses in consciousness and/or confusion.	Periodic medical updates may be required at discretion of DMV.	YES

COLORADO	No fixed period of time	Physician certification of fitness to drive must be submitted. Applicant must disclose a physical disability that would cause a lapse of consciousness.	Periodic medical updates may be required at discretion of DMV.	NO
CONNECTICUT	No fixed period of time	Physician certification of fitness to drive must be submitted. Licensing determination is made following receipt of required medical forms from the treating physician that is reviewed by the DMV and the Medical Advisory Board.	Periodic medical updates may be required at discretion of DMV.	NO
DELAWARE	No fixed period of time	A person with epilepsy must submit a certificate from their physician stating that their epilepsy is under sufficient control to permit them to safely operate a motor vehicle. If not, license restrictions are put in place.	Annual reviews are required.	Yes for events with loss of consciousness

DISTRICT OF COLUMBIA	12 months	Physician certification of fitness to drive must be submitted. Following a 5-year seizure free period, applicants are required to sign an affidavit that they have been seizure free and no further reports are then required. Restricted licenses are available.	Medical updates are required annually until seizure free for a full 5 years.	NO
FLORIDA	6 months, with doctor's recommen-dation	Physician certification of fitness to drive must be submitted. The Medical Advisory Board will deny a license following a 6-month period of seizure freedom when factors make it unsafe for the applicant to drive. Following a 2-year period of seizure freedom, a physician's certificate is no longer required.	Periodic medical updates may be required at discretion of Medical Advisory Board.	NO

GEORGIA	6 months	Physician certification of fitness to drive must be submitted. Those with nocturnal epilepsy may obtain a limited license.	Periodic medical updates may be required at discretion of Medical Review Board	NO
HAWAII	6 months (some exceptions apply)	Physician certification of fitness to drive must be submitted. All medical information is reviewed by the Medical Advisory Board on a case-by-case basis.	Periodic medical updates may be required at discretion of DMV.	NO
IDAHO	No fixed period of time	Physician certification of fitness to drive must be submitted. Licenses are denied due to momentary or prolonged lapses of consciousness or control.	Periodic medical updates may be required at discretion of DMV.	NO

ILLINOIS	No fixed period of time	Applicant must sign a medical agreement each time the required physician medical report is submitted stating they have agreed to remain under the care of their physician and are compliant. This agreement also gives permission to their physician to report any change in their condition that would impair their ability to safely operate a motor vehicle.	Periodic medical updates may be required at discretion of the Medical Advisory Board.	NO
INDIANA	No fixed period of time	An individual with epilepsy will not be denied a license if they present a statement from a licensed physician stating that they are taking their antiseizure medication and are free from seizures while taking these medications. Restricted licenses may be imposed.	Periodic medical updates may be required at discretion of Medical Advisory Board.	NO

IOWA	6 months (some exceptions apply)	Physician certification of fitness to drive must be submitted. An individual will not need to wait the 6-month period if their seizures occur only at night, were the result of a medication change or a pattern of syncope.	Periodic medical updates are required after 6 months and then at the time of renewal.	NO
KANSAS	6 months (some exceptions apply)	Physician certification of fitness to drive must be submitted. A person with a controlled seizure disorder is not considered to have a disability unless the Medical Advisory Board finds that the applicant is likely to be a danger to themselves or to others.	Periodic medical updates are required each year until seizure free for 3 years.	NO

KENTUCKY	90 days	Upon application or renewal, a person with epilepsy must submit a physician's statement certifying that the epilepsy is controlled by medication, give a description of the medications with dosages, and include a personal statement by the physician that they are compliant. Restricted or probationary licenses are available but seldom used.	Periodic medical updates are required upon renewal.	NO
LOUISIANA	6 months, with doctor's recommen-dation	A physician's certificate detailing fitness to drive is required. This is waived upon license renewal, except for commercial licenses.	Periodic medical reports may be required at discretion of DMV.	NO

			NO
MAINE	3 months, possibly longer	Physician certification of fitness to drive must be submitted. If seizure free for 3 months and compliant with medication, a license may be issued. Difficult cases are reviewed by the Medical Advisory Board.	Periodic medical reports may be required at discretion of DMV.
MARYLAND	3 months (some exceptions apply)	Medical Advisory Board determines eligibility based on required medical reports by physician.	Periodic medical reports may be required at discretion of DMV. NO
MASSACHU-SETTS	6 months	Must submit a detailed physician's report with recommendation that the individual can safely drive.	Periodic medical reports may be required at discretion of DMV. NO

MICHIGAN	6 months (some exceptions apply) 12 months for a chauffer's license	Waiting period may be reduced or eliminated based upon a departmental review of the specific recommendations of a qualified physician or other information received. Restricted licenses are available.	Periodic medical reports may be required at discretion of DMV.	NO
MINNESOTA	6 months (some exceptions apply)	Physician certification of fitness to drive must be submitted. Unless physician requires otherwise, a person seizure free for 4 years must only report every 4 years.	Depending on circumstances, periodic medical reports may be required by the DMV as often as every 6 months.	NO
MISSISSIPPI	12 months	Physician certification of fitness to drive must be submitted. No exceptions to the 12 month waiting period are offered.	Periodic medical reports may be required at discretion of Medical Advisory Board.	NO

MISSOURI	6 months, with doctor's recommendation	Physician certification of fitness to drive must be submitted. Conditional license usually granted for one year, followed by verification that applicant remains seizure free.	Periodic medical reports may be required at discretion of DMV.	NO
MONTANA	No fixed period of time; doctor's recommendation needed	Physician certification of fitness to drive must be submitted. Applicant must provide a brief description of condition that impairs or may impair ability to operate a motor vehicle safely. Determination made by DMV with consideration given to physician's opinion.	None required	NO

NEBRASKA	No fixed period of time	Physician certification of fitness to drive must be submitted. Applicants are given a thorough examination. DMV decisions are made on a case-by-case basis.	None required	NO
NEVADA	3 months (some exceptions apply)	Physician's medical report required for initial application or renewal. Information reviewed and determination made on a case-by-case basis by the DMV. Difficult cases are reviewed by the Medical Advisory Board.	Periodic medical reports may be required by the DMV every year for 3 years.	YES
NEW HAMPSHIRE	12 months or less (some exceptions apply)	Physician certification of fitness to drive must be submitted. Waiting period may be reduced if physician certifies seizures are not likely to continue.	None required	NO

NEW JERSEY	12 months (some exceptions apply); with neurological disorders committee recommendation	Licensing determinations are made by the Neurological Disorder Committee and are based on required medical records submitted by the applicant and his/her physician.	Medical updates must be submitted every 6 months for the first 2 years and every year thereafter.	YES
NEW MEXICO	12 months (some exceptions apply); with recommendation of Medical Advisory Board	Licensing determinations are made by the Medical Advisory Board and are based on required medical records submitted by the applicant and his/her physician. Probationary or restricted licenses are available.	Periodic medical reports may be required at discretion of Medical Advisory Board.	NO
NEW YORK	12 months (some exceptions apply)	Physician certification of fitness to drive must be submitted. Each case is reviewed individually. Restricted licenses are not available.	Periodic medical reports may be required at discretion of DMV.	NO

NORTH CAROLINA	6-12 months (some exceptions apply)	Physician certification of fitness to drive must be submitted. DMV Medical Advisor determines licensing eligibility based on special circumstances and on a case-by-case basis. Treatment compliance is also considered.	Periodic medical reports required annually unless DMV determines it is not necessary.	NO
NORTH DAKOTA	6 months; restricted license available after 3 months (some exceptions apply)	Applicant and physician must submit a sworn statement that individual has been seizure free for 6 months. Reduction in waiting period offered after 3 months with special circumstances. Restricted licenses available.	Periodic medical reports required annually for at least 3 years.	NO

			NO
OHIO	No fixed period of time	Physician certification of fitness to drive must be submitted. Applicant must swear to being seizure free and/or free from any similarly impairing condition. Falsifying this information could result in criminal prosecution. Restricted licenses are available.	Periodic medical reports required every 6 months or yearly until person is seizure free for 5 years.
OKLAHOMA	6 months (some exceptions apply)	Physician certification of fitness to drive must be submitted. An incident or portion of time involving altered consciousness and/or loss of body control requires the 6-month waiting period.	Periodic medical reports required at discretion of Department of Public Safety.	NO

OREGON	3 months (some exceptions apply)	Physician certification of fitness to drive must be submitted. A Certificate of Medical Eligibility is required assuring that any current medical condition does not impair ability to drive. Medical criteria guidelines outlined for the Driver Medical Certification Program are followed.	Periodic medical reports may be required at discretion of DMV.	YES
PENNSYLVANIA	6 months (some exceptions apply)	The seizure free period may be waived following a review of required information provided by the physician to the Medical Advisory Board.	Periodic medical reports may be required at discretion of Medical Advisory Board.	YES
PUERTO RICO	No fixed period of time	Physician certification of fitness to drive must be submitted. Restricted licenses are available.	Periodic medical reports may be required at discretion of Medical Advisory Board.	NO

RHODE ISLAND	18 months or less (some exceptions at discretion of DMV)	Physician certification of fitness to drive must be submitted.	Periodic medical reports may be required at discretion of DMV.	NO
SOUTH CAROLINA	6 months	Physician certification of fitness to drive must be submitted. Probationary licenses are not available.	Periodic medical reports are required at 6 months and then annually for 3 years.	NO
SOUTH DAKOTA	6-12 months or less. (some exceptions apply with doctor's recommen-dation)	Physician certification of fitness to drive must be submitted that includes that the individual's epilepsy is controlled by medication and that the applicant is continuing to take their medication. Restricted licenses are available.	Medical reports required every 6 months until seizure free for 1 year.	NO

			NO
TENNESSEE	6 months	Both the Medical Advisory Board and the physician must agree that the individual is safe to drive a motor vehicle.	Periodic medical reports may be required at discretion of Medical Advisory Board.
TEXAS	6 months (some exceptions apply)	Physician certification of fitness to drive must be submitted that includes information about the patient's compliance with medication, freedom from sleep deprivation and non-use of alcohol.

Restricted or probationary licenses are not available. | Periodic medical reports may be required at discretion of Medical Advisory Board.

NO |
| **UTAH** | 3 months (some exceptions apply) | Physician certification of fitness to drive must be submitted.

Driving restrictions, such as time of day, location, and speed, may be imposed at the recommendation of the treating physician. | Periodic medical reports may be required at discretion of Medical Advisory Board.

NO |

VERMONT	No fixed period of time	Physician certification of fitness to drive must be submitted. Must receive medical evaluation from Commissioner. Restricted licenses are sometimes available.	Periodic medical reports may be required at discretion of Medical Advisory Board.	NO
VIRGINIA	6 months (some exceptions apply)	Physician certification of fitness to drive must be submitted. Applicant must prove they are free from a medical condition that "will prevent him or her from exercising reasonable and ordinary control over a motor vehicle."	Periodic medical reports may be required at discretion of Medical Advisory Board.	NO
WASHINGTON	6 months (some exceptions apply)	Waiting period may be waived following physical examination and/or physician statement supporting ability to safely operate a motor vehicle.	Periodic medical reports may be required the by the Medical Advisory Board.	NO

WEST VIRGINIA	12 months (some exceptions apply)	Physician certification of fitness to drive must be submitted. Difficult cases are reviewed by the Medical Advisory Board. Restricted licenses are available that place limitation son time, day or travel distance.	Periodic medical reports may be required the by the Medical Advisory Board.	NO
WISCONSIN	3 months, with doctor's recommen–dation	Physician certification of fitness to drive must be submitted. No exemptions or restricted licenses are available.	Periodic medical reports may be required the by the Medical Advisory Board.	NO
WYOMING	3 months (some exceptions apply)	If a written medical statement from qualified medical professional states that a person experiences a loss, interruption, or lapse of consciousness and/or motor function, a license may be denied or revoked. Daytime licenses are available for persons with only nocturnal seizures.	Periodic medical reports may be required the by the Medical Advisory Board.	NO

Please note:

Law making is dynamic process; thus driving laws are subject to change whenever state legislatures convene. Please contact your local DMV for the most up-to-date information. You can also visit the following website for the most current verification of the driving laws in your state:

- **Driving and Travel: Driver Information by State** http://www.epilepsyfoundation.org/resources/drivingandtravel.cfm

APPENDIX 3
SYMPTOMATIC PARTIAL EPILEPSY BY LOBE

Partial epilepsy arises from the outer layer of the brain – the cortex – which is divided into four lobes: temporal, frontal, parietal, and occipital. Partial seizures cause the disruption of normal functioning in a part of the brain, usually in just one of the lobes (as opposed to seizures that involve the whole brain). Since each of these lobes govern different functions, the seizures that arise from specific lobes will cause certain specific symptoms.

Also, seizures can either "turn on" brain cells, activating their function, or "turn off" brain cells, disabling function. So a seizure in the visual center of the brain (occipital lobe) could either turn on the brain cells, causing visual hallucinations, or turn them off, causing temporary blindness.

Let's take a look at the functions of the lobes and the characteristic features of partial seizures that occur in each of them.

TEMPORAL LOBE EPILEPSY

The temporal lobe is the most common location for partial epilepsy. Functions of the temporal lobe include memory, smell, hearing, automatic behavior, autonomic function (heart rate, digestion, perspiration, etc.) and the understanding of speech. Thus, the seizure will produce symptoms that affect these areas, such as:

- déjà vu (a sense that something has happened before)

- jamais vu (a sense that something has never happened before, or being unfamiliar with a familiar situation or person)

- a smell

- confusion and inability to interact with the surrounding environment

- a sensation of fear

- auditory hallucinations such as ringing in the ears or hearing music

- no memory of the event

- automatic movements (automatisms) such as lip smacking or picking at clothes

- dystonia (fixed posturing of an arm or leg)

- Understanding of speech if the dominant hemisphere is involved (left hemisphere in right handed individuals and left or right hemisphere in left handed ones)

Temporal lobe seizures can occur during the day or night. There is no typical trigger. Four out of ten persons with temporal lobe epilepsy will not respond to medical treatment and may be candidates for epilepsy surgery.

FRONTAL LOBE EPILEPSY

Frontal lobe epilepsy is the second most common location for partial epilepsy. The largest lobe of the brain, the frontal lobe is involved in control of movements, planning, social skills and expression of speech. Symptoms of frontal lobe epilepsy include:

- abnormal movements, which can range from rhythmic jerking of one extremity to bizarre complicated movements involving multiple extremities (e.g., bicycling movements of the legs or running).

- a sustained, unnatural turning of the head and eyes to one side (head and eye deviation)

- expression of speech (left hemisphere in right handed individuals and left or right hemisphere in left handed ones)
- a smell
- staring off the space

Frontal lobe seizures frequently occur at nighttime. Sometimes the movements can be so erratic that they are confused with non-epileptic events. Frontal lobe seizures tend to be briefer than other types of partial seizures.

PARIETAL LOBE EPILEPSY

The parietal lobe controls the feelings of touch. While relatively rare, seizures in this lobe cause:

- numbness on one side of the body

- tingling on one side of the body

Seizures that begin in the parietal lobe may spread rapidly to other regions of the brain, mimicking the signs and symptoms of other forms of partial epilepsy. Parietal seizures can happen either during the day or night, and there is no particular trigger.

OCCIPITAL LOBE EPILEPSY

The occipital lobe contains the visual center of the brain. Symptoms of occipital lobe epilepsy include:

- simple visual phenomena, such as seeing flashing lights

- complex visual phenomena, such as seeing a flag that isn't there or a brief sequence of images like a movie.

- the head and eyes may suddenly turn to one side.

- nausea

- headaches

- Temporary loss of vision

Like parietal seizures, occipital seizures can spread rapidly to other regions of the brain, mimicking the signs and symptoms of other forms of partial epilepsy. Occipital seizures can occur during the day or night and, in rare cases, may be triggered by flashing lights (photosensitivity).

APPENDIX 4
MEDICATIONS THAT CAN INCREASE POTENTIAL OF HAVING SEIZURES

Certain medications that you might be taking for other health conditions can contribute to your risk of experiencing seizures, either while you're actively taking them or when you're withdrawing from them. These medications can be divided into four categories according to the likelihood of an increased risk (definite, possible, possible slight, and possible very slight), with a fifth category containing medications that have reported association with seizures but the accompanying risk is unknown.

Take a look through these lists to see if you are taking any of the medications listed. If so, be sure to tell your doctor immediately.

DEFINITE INCREASE IN RISK (>0.1%)		
Bupropion	Wellbutrin®	>300 mg/day
Clozapine	Clozaril®, Fazaclo®	
Flurazepam	Dalmane®	In withdrawal
theophylline	Uniphyl®	
Tramadol	Ultram ®	

POSSIBLE MODERATE INCREASE IN RISK
(>0.01% but <0.1%)

4-aminopyridine	Fampridine ®	
alprazolam	Xanax ®	In withdrawal
amitriptyline	Elavil ®	
amoxapine	Moxadil ®	
aripiprazole	Abilify ®	
atomexietine	Strattera ®	
buspirone	BuSpar ®	
cefixime	Suprax ®	
citalopram	Celexa ®	
clomipramine	Anafranil ®	
cyclobenzaprine	Amrix®, Flexeril®	
duloxetine	Cymbalta ®	
epoetin	Epogen ®	
fluoxetine	Prozac ®	
inteferon beta-1a	Avonex®	
inteferon beta-1b	Rebif®, Betaseron ®	
memantine	Namenda®	
meropenem	Merrem ®	
mitoxantrone	Novantrone®	
ofloxacin	Floxin ®	
olanzapine	Zyprexa ®	
paroxetine	Paxil ®	
protriptyline	Vivactil ®	
quietapine	Seroquel ®	
risperidone	Risperdal ®	
sertraline	Zoloft ®	
sibutramine	Meridia ®	
torsemide	Demadex ®	
trihexyphenidyl	Artane ®	
venlafaxine	Effexor ®	
ziprasidone	Geodon ®	

POSSIBLE SLIGHT INCREASE IN RISK
(<0.01% but >0.001%)

clomiphene	Clomid ®	
dantrolene	Dantrium ®	
desipramine	Norpramin ®	
doxepin	Sinequan ®	In withdrawal
escitalopram	Lexapro ®	
etoposide	Vepesid ®	
glatiramer	Copaxone ®	
haloperidol	Haldol ®	
mirazapine	Remeron®	
nortriptyline	Pamelor ®	
oxytocin	Pitocin ®	
Percodan	Percocet ®	
thiothixene	Navane ®	
tizanidine	Zanaflex ®	
trifluperazine	Stelazine ®	

POSSIBLE VERY SLIGHT INCREASE IN RISK
(<0.001%)

baclofen	Lioresal ®	In withdrawal
busulfan	Myleran ®	
chlorambucil	Leukeran ®	
chlorpromazin	Thorazine ®	
diphenhydramine	Benadryl ®	In withdrawal
hydroxyzine	Atarax®, Vistaril®	In withdrawal
lorazepam	Ativan ®	In withdrawal
molindone	Moban ®	
ondansetron	Zofran ®	
phenylpropanolamine	Dexatrim®	
terbutaline	Terbutaline®	

REPORTED ASSOCIATION WITH SEIZURE, BUT UNKNOWN INCREASE IN RISK		
Alcohol		In withdrawal
almotriptan	Axert ®	
aminophylline	Truphylline ®	
Amphetamines	Adderal ®	
amphotericin	B Amphotec ®	
atorvastatin	Lipitor ®	
azathioprine	Imuran ®	
benztropine	Cogentin ®	
bromocriptine	Parlodel ®	
bupivicaine	Marcaine ®	
cabergoline	Dostinex ®	
caffeine	Cafcit ®	
captopril	Capoten®	
carisoprodol	Soma ®	In withdrawal
carvedilol	Coreg ®	
cefepime	Maxipime ®	
cefotetan	Cefotan ®	
ceftazidime	Fortaz®, Tazidime ®	
cefuroxime	Zinacef ®	
cephalexin	Keflex ®	
chloroquine	Aralen ®	
ciprofloxacin	Cipro ®	
cisplatinum	Cisplatin ®	
clonazepam	Klonopin®	In withdrawal
clorazepate	Tranxene ®	In withdrawal
cocaine		
cyclophosphamide	Cytoxan ®	
cyclosporin	Sandimmune®, Gengraf ®	
dexmethylphenidate	Focalin ®	
dexoamphetamine	Dexedrine ®	
dextroamphetamine	Dexedrine ®	

diazepam	Valium ®	In withdrawal
dicyclomine	Bentyl ®	
donepezil	Aricept ®	
doripenem	Doribax ®	
doxorubicin	Adriamycin ®	
dronabinol	Marinol ®	
efavirenz	Sustiva ®	
enfluraneketamine	Enflurane ®	
entacapone	Comtan ®	
estazolam	ProSom ®	In withdrawal
estrogen	Premarin ®	
eszopiclone	Lunesta ®	In withdrawal
fentanyl	Duragesic ®	
fluphenazine	Prolixin ®	
fluvastatin	Lescol XL®	
ganciclovir	Cytovene ®	
gemifloxacin	Factive ®	
Ginkgo biloba		
imipenim/cilastin	Primaxin ®	
indomethacin	Indocin ®	
Isoniazid	Nydrazid ®	
ivermectin	Stromectol ®	
ketorolac	Toradol ®	
levofloxacin	Levaquin ®	
lidocaine	Xylocaine ®	
lindane	Agrocide ®	
linezolid	Zyvox ®	
lithium	Lithobid®	
lomefloxacin	Maxaquin ®	
loxapine	Loxitane ®	
mefenamic acid	Ponstel ®	
mefloquin	Larium ®	
meperidine	Demerol ®	
mephobarbital	Mebaral ®	In withdrawal

methocarbamol	Robaxin ®	
methotrexate	Trexall ®	
methylphenidate	Concerta®, Ritalin ®	
metronidazole	Flagyl ®	
modafinil	Provigil ®	
montelukast	Singulair ®	
moxifloxacin	Avelox ®	
mycophenolate	CellCept®	
nalidixic acid	Negram ®	
oxybutynin	Ditropan ®	
oxycodone	Oxycontin ®	
oxymorphone	Opana ®	
pentazocine	Talwin ®	
phenobarbital	Luminal ®	In withdrawal
pimozide	Orap ®	
pramipexole	Mirapex®	
prednisone	Deltason ®	
primidone	Mysoline ®	In withdrawal
procaine	Novocain ®	
promethazine	Phenergan ®	
propoxyphene	Darvon ®	
rameltron	Rozerem ®	In withdrawal
rasagiline	Azilect ®	
rivastigmine	Exelon ®	
ropinerole	Requip ®	
selegiline	Eldeprel ®	
sildenafil	Viagra ®	
sodium oxybate	Xyrem ®	
sumatriptan	Imitrex ®	
tacrine	Cognex ®	
tacrolimus	Prograf®	
tadalafil	Cialis ®	
temazepam	Restoril ®	In withdrawal
temozolomide	Temodar ®	

thalidomide	Thalomid ®	
thioridazine	Mellaril ®	
ticlopidine	Ticlid ®	
tinidazole	Tindamax®	
tolcapone	Tasmar ®	
tolterodine	Detrol-LA®	
tranylcypromine	Parnate ®	
triazolam	Halcion ®	In withdrawal
valacyclovir	Valtrex ®	
valsartan	Diovan ®	
vardenafil	Levitra ®	
vincristine	Oncovin ®	
zaleplon	Sonata ®	In withdrawal
zanamivir	Relenza ®	
ziconotide	Prialt ®	
zidovudine	Retrovir capsules®	
zolpidem	Ambien ®	In withdrawal

INDEX

20057703R00188

Made in the USA
Lexington, KY
17 January 2013